7 Keys to AWESOME Health

Jana L. Fortner, N.D.

ISBN-10:1475128347
ISBN-13:978-1475128345

DEDICATION

This book is dedicated to my family, those of us together now, and those who wait for us beyond this world; they left us too soon. I wish I had known then what I know now. My family is everything to me.

Without my husband's support, encouragement, and untiring enthusiasm for my efforts, I would not be where I am today in any sense. My children never cease to inspire me, amaze me, and believe in me; they give me the strength to keep trying for the future we all want to build. My mother is the soul of love and patience and faith, without whom I doubt I would be anywhere at all. I thank God for all of you.

Eternal thanks to all of you.

TABLE OF CONTENTS

Disclaimer

None of the information offered in this book or on our website or contained in any material presented by Dr. Fortner or the Nutritional Health Education Center is intended to diagnose or treat disease; nor is it to be considered as medical advice or a replacement for medical advice. It is presented for educational purposes only. All risks associated with actions you choose to take after reading this material are your sole responsibility and no liability will be assumed by Dr. Fortner or the Nutritional Health Education Center. As with all other information from any source, it is your responsibility to exercise sound judgment and discretion before you act.

If you are taking prescription medication, please be aware that it is not advisable to discontinue it or reduce it without a doctor's supervision. If you have a medical condition, it is also unwise to begin an exercise regimen without a doctor's advice. Serious harm may result from such actions.

Introduction

What Is Health? What Is Healing?

According to the New Webster's Dictionary, health is merely the absence of disease. The dictionary says that disease is an impairment of the functioning of a system of the body or an organ or part. This book is for people who believe health is more than that. There is a lot of ground between visible, measurable, symptomatic disease and robust, optimal health.

Let's create a more useful definition. I believe health is your personal best physically, mentally, and emotionally. Health is when everything is working right—you're firing on all eight cylinders. You're in factory condition, not just satisfactory condition. You're able to function fully and your defenses are strong enough to keep you that way.

One of those natural functions is to repair damage that occurs in the process of life. So if health means being fully functional, then healing is the automatic, internal process your body goes through to repair damage and restore that normal function. We have self-healing bodies—very awesome when you think about it.

If you've ever cut your finger and noticed its daily progress as it returns to normal without your or your doctor's assistance, you know that this capacity for repair, for healing, is built into every cell in your body. The best part is that it happens just the same on the inside where you can't see it.

These common-sense points of view represent a shift for many people in our culture. How many people do you know who need prescription medications every day to force their bodies to function anywhere near normal? How many of them would say that they are basically healthy?

How many medical doctors would describe patients on medications as "healthy," and how many patients with parts missing altogether such as a gall bladder, appendix, a section of intestine, or even a kidney are routinely referred to as healthy while no effort whatsoever is made to restore the function that was lost?

A healthy body will have enough energy to get through a normal days' work with enough left over to enjoy the evening. A healthy body will not get colds or infections every year. Healthy people don't have headaches, acid indigestion, constipation, declining vision, and high blood pressure. It is not a necessary part of aging to be aching and tired all the time. The bottom line is this: healthy people aren't sick!

Are you ready to raise the standard? Let's do that where health and healing are concerned right now by realizing that:

- If you require medication to force your body to accomplish its normal daily tasks, you are NOT healthy.
- If you are suffering physically or mentally, you are NOT healthy.
- If you can't pursue your purpose or passion in life because of your body, you are NOT healthy.

Knowledge is power, and responsibility is a position of power. Only when you acknowledge that you are not healthy can you begin to move away from that place; only when you accept responsibility for your own health can you take the first step.

If you are dissatisfied with your health and your health care right now, I want to congratulate you! You are in a great place where tremendous opportunity is within your grasp right now. Use your dissatisfaction as the rocket fuel it takes to move you to a higher orbit in life.

There are seven exciting truths about how the body works that everyone needs to understand:

1. Your body is made entirely of cells which routinely die and get replaced.
2. Every year you pretty much grow a brand new body (see #1).
3. This year's new body is made of whatever you ate last year.
4. Your body does not make mistakes. It always does the best it can with what you give it.
5. Your body was designed to repair itself—no matter what's wrong.
6. There is nothing you can't make better by giving your body what it needs.

7.   There is NO drug, and there is NO doctor of any kind anywhere on earth that can heal anything, ever. We can be helpful, but ultimately, the body MUST heal itself—there are NO exceptions.

If you are like most people, this list has generated some questions, maybe even some challenges in your mind. Are these things true or is this just hype? Asking good questions is that first step in learning something new—and if you've got some, that's great—actually, that's healthy!

After years of study, personal experience, and seeing clients who have successfully transformed their health and their lives, I have found that there are seven major factors that almost entirely determine our health—and they are ALL things we have control over. My mission is to teach people how to manage these seven factors to make the most of their God-given potential for good health by allowing their bodies to heal. I want to end as much suffering as possible for as many people as possible. When you control the 7 Keys to AWESOME Health, you control your own destiny.

How to use this book

What are the seven things within your control that largely determine your health status? They are Attitude, Water, Elimination, Sleep, Oxygen, Maximum nutrition, and Exercise. These are the keys you need to unlock your AWESOME health potential and live your life to the fullest.

This book was designed to walk you through these 7 Keys one chapter, and one key, at a time. It's best to read through the chapters and take on the challenges in order. Some of the chapters are set up like workshops to take you through a transformational process step by step and there are summaries at the end of each chapter for quick reference. In Appendix A, there is a summary of useful lists and acronyms used in the book to help you organize and retain the concepts taught in each chapter.

There is no need to live in fear for your future. Good health is a basic human right. You deserve it, and you can have it. If you want to be healthy for the rest of your life, I challenge you to take responsibility now for everything your life is and everything you want it to be. No one can do it for you, but you are not alone. I am honored to help you on your journey.

Chapter 1: Attitude Is Everything

If you're looking for a book full of references to the latest scientific studies, you haven't found it. Building your health program around the latest news is confusing, expensive, and exhausting—I know because I've been there. I want to arm you with knowledge and common sense so you can decide for yourself whether you are hearing the truth or not—not just for today, but for a lifetime. Studies are frequently engineered and financed by people who have a financial interest in the outcome. How can you trust that?

Using what you already know by experience, some basic facts that are beyond dispute, and even a few simple experiments you can do yourself, we can figure out what it takes to be well. Wouldn't confidence in your health program feel great? My basic philosophy is that health wasn't meant to be hard. Philosophy is a very important piece of every puzzle because it determines how you approach problems; it's all about your attitude.

This book is about empowering you to take charge of your own health, your own destiny. This is your life! It should be exciting, right? "Attitude is everything" doesn't sound very exciting, but it truly is. Sometimes eloquence and simplicity are one.

This isn't a book about religion, but there is no better analogy for the significance of attitude in the journey toward health than a story from I Kings chapter 5 in the Bible about a man named Naaman who suffered from the deadly skin disease, leprosy. He was told by Elijah the prophet to dip himself in the muddy Jordan River seven times in order to be made well. Now Naaman was not excited. In fact, he was furious. Naaman's expectations (attitude) were causing him trouble. You can probably relate to how he must have felt. He had made a long, difficult journey to reach this prophet and along the way he had lots of time to imagine the encounter.

By the time he reached the prophet's house, he had some very concrete expectations built up. He thought the prophet would come out and do amazing and interesting things. It would be quite an occasion and the whole process would be spectacular. Now he was bitterly disappointed. No show at all. In fact, the prophet didn't even bother to come out of his house! He sent a servant to tell Naaman what to do. What a blow to the ego! With his expectations thus severely violated, he was ready to pack up and go home. Why should he dip himself in some nasty river? That would never work anyway…

As he prepared to leave, his own servant stopped him. The servant said, in essence, "You were prepared to do something really awful, really hard, even weird, so why be disappointed that it's so simple? You've come this far, why not have a little faith and give it a shot?"

Naaman went down into the river six times—and there was no change. How must he have felt when he was about to go in for the seventh time? Nervous, perhaps. Braced for disappointment, surely. Yet he had enough faith to follow through with that seventh trip under the water. He didn't see any reason for this to work, but he had enough faith to try. After the seventh dunking, he came up with skin like a baby. He was a very happy man. Suddenly, what moments before seemed dull and even stupid now felt like an awesome miracle.

When you feel yourself getting well, it feels like a miracle—no matter how simple your method of healing was. Some people are so stuck on wanting a wonder pill, they can't believe in anything else. They can't try anything else. That's a shame.

In this book I want to give you seven tasks to complete to recover your health. These 7 Keys are not amazing. They are not original. There will be no fireworks, and probably no magazine cover stories. But these simple things do work. Don't dismiss them because they are simple; instead, have enough faith to try. You can't say this won't work because you know you've never applied all 7 Keys correctly; probably not all in the same year, never mind in the same day—every day!

If you honestly and diligently apply the principles in this book for at least 30 days—without cheating—and you are not feeling better than you have in a long time that will be amazing. I think you will be very happy at the end of 30 days. If you stick with it for a year, you'll have a new lease on life. If you stay with it for life, you'll be much more likely to live a very long life free of disease, medication, and trouble.

As a man thinks in his heart, so is he...

This is a great saying, full of truth. Modern science has only just begun to understand it. To illustrate certain aspects of this truism, consider a man in a third world country. His home is in a war zone. His dwelling is barely a shack and all his possessions could be carried in a sack on his back—and they have been, three times in the past six months.

He has lived on one meal per day for as long as his country's war has lasted and there is no crop to look forward to in the coming year at all. He has one cooking pot, his knife, a thin blanket, and one change of clothing. Every night he prays for safety for one more day. Every morning he wakes up and tearfully thanks God for making him such a rich man. Huh?

He is rich in his own eyes because his wife is lying next to him on one side, and his children are all alive and well on the other. His parents are asleep in the next tent over. He is the only man from his village whose family is still intact; the only man who has not yet buried a wife or a child. He IS rich. That is his reality.

It is largely a matter of perspective and values, but it is no less true. Rich, happy, blessed, or miserable are not objective realities—they are subjective emotions. If you argued the point with him, he would tell you that your priorities are skewed from easy living; that you don't value what really matters in life. Your own expectations, your own requirements, are your freedom or your prison.

My question for you is this: Which of you experienced more happiness today? The man in the illustration, or you? It is a question worth pondering because you don't need a scientific study to tell you that whether or not you are happy is tightly linked with your health. You already know that when you're really happy you feel better. I can tell you, as can most spiritual leaders from history and the present, that happiness and gratitude are actually one and the same.

Of course, it is very important for you to be aware of whatever situation led you to purchase this book. You must tell yourself the truth about your health, but you must not overlook the good in your life. Everything is not bad. You are blessed that your eyes still work—you are reading. If someone is reading to you, you are blessed to have such a friend.

Why this emphasis on the positive? There is a very important principle that all great leaders and coaches know: where your focus is, your power is also. Your attention is a form of energy, an active form that causes growth and change. Your mind directs this energy and whatever "facts" you present to yourself on a daily basis become your view of the truth. For example, if you are concerned that you might feel sick at your stomach, and you focus on your stomach—looking for that feeling and thinking about whether or not it's there, chances are that pretty soon you will begin to feel sick.

If you believe your coworker, Joe, doesn't like you, you will begin to watch him—looking for evidence of treachery. You will interpret his actions through a lens of suspicion, and everything he says and does will take on a sinister hue. Soon you will have ample evidence to support your hypothesis that Joe has it in for you.

Your brain is a powerful entity which exists to bring into reality that which you think about all the time. If you tell your brain you are fat, it will supply you with a wide variety of activities that will support that *chosen* identity.

If you want to test this theory, ask your mind a question. Why am I such a nice person? If you honestly try, your mind will generate a list for you. Now, ask yourself another question. Why am I such a jerk? Got another list, right? Ask a good question, get a good answer. Ask a bad question... Your brain serves your mind. It's not picky about what it works on.

If you tell yourself every day that you *are* a "heart attack looking for a place to happen," or you *are* a cancer victim, you *are* fat, or you *will always have* indigestion, you will bring these things about far more readily than someone else who does not label himself this way. We choose our own identity, our labels, our destiny.

I am here to tell you right now that you *are not* a disease carrier—you are a person; you are (your name here), and nothing else. It is not healthy to link your identity—your existence—with something unhealthy or undesirable. Therefore...

1. Reclaim your identity: Step 1 in the journey to regain your health is to reclaim your identity.

You must let go of all other descriptions of yourself and your situation that don't support the life you want to lead. Be yourself, and nothing else. No labels. When you do this, really do it, you'll feel a sense of wholeness and freedom and things will feel fresh and new. That's a very good state for healing to occur in; never forget that feeling. It's the perfect starting point.

Once you have reacquainted yourself with who you really are and you have acknowledged what's in your life at this moment that you want to change, you must begin to take actions that will bring change. Remember that you are not your body, your health, your habits, or your circumstances. There is nothing wrong with...you. You...are designed, and wanted, by God. God doesn't make mistakes; though people often do.

Remember that the actions you have taken in your life leading up to this day have brought you to this point physically, mentally, spiritually etc. You do reap what you sow. That is the good—and the bad—news. You are reaping what you sowed in prior years, but you still have the power to control what you plant for next season. The seeds are in your hands. Only the seeds you plant will grow; not the ones you leave in the bag.

2. Standards: Step 2 is to decide what you want and state that clearly for your own benefit.

Write down your standards and share them with someone who will support you and help you be accountable for living the life you choose. This is not the same as "New Year's resolutions," which are lofty goals we abandon immediately. These are standards for living that redefine who you are and what your purpose is in life. As you review these statements, preferably daily, you become reacquainted with your purpose, and it strengthens your resolve.

Some examples of good standards include:

- I am committed to my own health.
- I will do whatever it takes to overcome my health obstacles.
- Excellent health is not optional, it is required.

Write down one or more standards for yourself that will inspire, challenge, and encourage you to do what you need to do. Post this in a place that will ensure that you see it several times daily, and read it aloud each time. Over a period of weeks, you will be able to realign your focus and assimilate this into your identity even when you are not looking at it. It takes time; don't give up.

3. Reasons to change: Step 3 is to get a clear vision of your reasons for making a change.

Why do you need to live? Why do you need to be well? Who is depending on you? Who would suffer without you? What do you want to contribute to the world? To your family? What do you want to do for yourself? What do you want to experience? What do you want to become?

You need to know why. Why are you willing to do things differently than you have before; why are you willing to sow different seeds now? You need to be aware of your reasons and be in touch with them on a daily basis. Making diet and lifestyle changes can be hard. You need strong reasons or you'll quit. The supports of the bridge between where you are and where you want to be are built with "musts" not with "maybes." Why must you live by these standards? Why now?

The path of least resistance is usually also the path of least reward. Letting yourself off the hook today generally means swallowing the hook tomorrow. For those of you who have never been fishing, a fish hooked in the mouth is easily released with minimal harm. A fish that stays on the line too long will swallow the hook and you'll make a bloody mess trying to free him.

There is no escape from the consequences of things you don't do. If you want a harvest, you have to get out the hoe and plant the seed. Where your health is concerned, no one—not even the best doctor in the world—can do this for you. All they can do is try to remove the hook.

Now take your standards and add your reasons:

- I am committed to my own health, because I want to know what it feels like to be my best. I deserve to be healthy.

- I will do whatever it takes to overcome health obstacles, so that I can be there for myself, my spouse, my children, and my grandchildren.

- Excellent health is not optional, it is required, because I have a lot to give to this world and I want to be able to give it 100%.

4. Goals: Step 4 is to set goals that will help you achieve your purpose.

Regardless of the ultimate desired outcome, learning about the subject is always a powerful first goal. Finishing this book, and perhaps even reading it a second time, would be a very appropriate first goal.

Having accomplished that, you will need other, more tangible goals - the planks on your bridge. The possibilities are almost endless.

Good: I will lose 20 pounds by the end of this year.

Good: I will give up _____.

Good: I will begin exercising _____ times per week for _____ minutes.

Best! I will correct all seven key areas, one per week/month.

More is not always better, and so it is with standards, reasons, and goals. Keeping this document short allows you to better control your focus. If it fits on an index card; so much the better. Buy yourself a greeting card with a message that compassionately inspires you and write it there if you like. Either way, carry it with you and read it often.

Laser focus

Consider a laser beam. If it is scattered over an area the size of a coffee can, it will be much less powerful than if the beam is reduced to an area the size of a pin head. An intensely focused beam will quickly bore a hole through even the hardest surface. That's what you need now—laser focus. It doesn't have to be 24/7. If you give your full attention to the matter of your health, even if only for a short time each day, you will surely have a breakthrough.

One last, but extremely important point is this: above all else, love yourself. Do not use this book to beat yourself up or show yourself the ways in which you have failed to protect your health in the past. We all make decisions for reasons. Sometimes we understand the reasons and sometimes we don't, but we do try to do well for ourselves. We do try to protect ourselves.

Compensation—what it means for your health

Sometimes it feels like your own body is trying to kill you, but that is not true. It has a reason for what it does and true malfunctions are rare, if they exist at all. Most of what we perceive as malfunction is actually compensation—your body's attempts to do the best it can under the circumstances it has to live with. Compensation can be painful, inconvenient, and even dangerous, but it is always better than the alternatives or your body would not have chosen it.

For example, suppose you have been drinking nothing but coffee and pop for years. Given that these liquids are actually mildly dehydrating agents, and you didn't drink enough even of these unhealthy choices, your body is now seriously dehydrated. Your body has been rationing water and conserving water, unbeknownst to you, for the first few years, but it's ability to do this has been exhausted and your blood volume has been reduced—due strictly to lack of water. Your doctor finds that your recent headaches are caused by the high blood pressure you have "suddenly and inexplicably" developed.

Why did your body betray you in this fashion? It didn't. The only way your body could continue to provide your brain with a sufficient blood supply to keep you gainfully employed was to raise your blood pressure—like putting your thumb over the end of a trickling water hose to boost the spray to reach that last distant plant in the garden. The headache and higher pressure reading were things your body was willing to endure in order to avoid passing out and experiencing brain damage from lack of blood flow. If you don't correct the problem, your blood pressure may crash and you might pass out from chronic low blood volume. This scenario is simplified and exaggerated to make a point: your body always does the best it can with what you give it. If you don't like the quality of life your body is giving you, consider what quality of life you're giving it!

Similarly in life, we always do the best we can with what we know, what we have, and what we feel. Maya Angelou said, "You did what you knew how to do, and when you knew better, you did better." The apostle Paul said, "Forgetting those things which are behind, I press on…" Taken together, these two come out like this: Don't worry about what happened before, learn and do better now. That is my advice to you. Don't look back and regret, look forward and do what you can, now.

The road to success is paved with many failures. The trick is to learn from them and do better. The only way you can ever really fail is to stop trying. If you fall short one day, get back on the horse the next. The best way to reach your goals is to keep riding until you get there.

Review

Key #1 Attitude is Everything

Attitude recovery plan:

Step 1: Reclaim your identity by letting go of labels. Be yourself and nothing else.

Step 2: Decide what you want and state that clearly for your own benefit.

Step 3: Get a clear vision of your reasons for making a change.

Step 4: Set goals that will help you achieve your purpose.

Step 5: Love yourself enough to keep riding until you get there.

Chapter 2: Water

You know who you are, you know what you want, you know why you want it, and in this chapter you have an opportunity to take all that insight and motivation you've found and use it to really make a difference in your health as you accept the challenge of mastering the second key to awesome health. You must optimize your water intake. Drinking water isn't very exciting, on the surface, but if you look a little deeper, there are many solid reasons to take firm hold of this key.

Positive uses of water in the body

According to James Balch, M.D., in *Prescription for Nutritional Healing*, "Water is an essential nutrient that is involved in every function of the body. It helps transport nutrients and waste products in and out of cells. It is necessary for all digestive, absorptive, circulatory, and excretory functions, as well as for the utilization of water-soluble vitamins. It is also needed for the maintenance of proper body temperature."[5]

If that description didn't stir your soul, let me put it another way. Your body cannot perform ANY of its vital functions without water. Water is a key component in the mass transportation system of the body. Like busses, trains, and planes carry things in and out of cities, the water in your body carries things where they need to go. If the mass transit systems shut down, the local economy is paralyzed. In the absence of water, many body systems are also seriously functionally impaired.

Have you ever seen a plant die from lack of water? Your body cells operate on principles very similar to plant cells. Just like the cells of the plant, your own cells can shrivel up, cease to function, and die from lack of water.

You can't even digest your food without water—you'd be surprised how many people taking drugs for indigestion are really suffering from dehydration. No vitamins, minerals, or anything else can be used by your body without water. Your body can't make energy efficiently without water. Because your blood is mostly water, the health of your arteries depends, in part, on your water supply, and you can't "clean house" without water, either.

Before we go any further, let's clarify the goal for this key. We want to drink adequate water while avoiding beverages that undermine the process of getting water into our cells. Water is good. Pop, coffee, black tea, and alcohol are harmful and need to be avoided if re-hydration is your goal. The caffeine in these drinks functions like a diuretic to take water out of your body. The amount of caffeine isn't enough to cause serious problems by itself, but there are so many other bad ingredients that the toxic load increases your need for good clean water to wash it all out. You don't need to take a big step in the wrong direction.

Understanding the function of water inside the body

Most experts would agree that a healthy human body is roughly 70% water. So where is all that water?

The body is made of cells, all of which contain fluid, which is mostly water. Imagine building something out of 100 trillion tiny sandwich bags of varying sizes full of water, and you get a strange, yet not inaccurate, view of your body. Imagine that some of the bags are squishy and full of oils while others are hard and full of proteins and minerals and you understand fat cells and bone cells.

Imagine that some of the bags are glued together to form hollow tubes through which more fluid, mostly water, can be channeled and you have your blood vessels. Add a pump, also made of bags, to move that fluid through the tubes and you've got a heart. There are other organs made of bags doing lots of other jobs, but you get the idea of where all the water is.

Just to give you some perspective, a cell is much larger than an atom or a molecule. Maybe that would be like comparing an RV to a golf ball. Your cells are obviously not made of plastic, though modern science is probably working feverishly somewhere to achieve that. They are made of a very complicated combination of molecules that are waterproof on one side and not on the other so that things can be moved, by chemistry and physics, in and out of the bag through tiny little portals without "unzipping" the whole bag and spilling everything. The portals are a little like the locks ships go through to get to the other side of a canal.

That's enough quasi-technical talk for you to appreciate the significance, at least on some level, of keeping those bags full. What will your imaginary creation look like if all the bags have only a little water in them? How will they function? You don't want your cells looking like raisins, you want nice plump grapes. Grapes look alive, raisins don't. You can appreciate the significance of the principle with regard to the wrinkles you would like to prevent or erase. As the cells dry out, the wrinkles deepen; as the cells plump up, the wrinkles cease to appear. Apply that principle to the entire body.

Toxicity and symptoms

Assuming you are not part of the tiny percentage of the population who are disabled due to a true genetic abnormality, there are two root causes of disease. This is a major point; don't miss it! The two causes for disease in the body are:

1. Toxicity

2. Deficiency

It's simple, but profound. Bodies function really well when they are not burdened by toxins, poisons that hinder our functioning, and when they are not lacking the basic elements they need to get their job done.

In toxicity, your body says, "Waiter, there's a fly in my soup." In deficiency, your body says, "I ordered that soup three hours ago, and it's still not here! I'm starving!"

We mention this here because water is needed to help clean out the body and to help bring nutrition into your cells. You can't get rid of wastes without adequate water, which explains why laxatives are perennial best-sellers in every pharmacy in America. To quote children's author J.K. Rowling, completely out of context, dehydration is a very big part of "the constipation sensation that's gripping the nation."[8]

Unfinished business

When we fail to drink enough water, the body's functions become altered chemically and physiologically in an effort to hold on to what little water we have. It's not unlike the city "drought plan" that goes into effect in late summer when rain is scarce. We can't wash the car, water the lawn, or play in the sprinklers for a few weeks because we need to save water.

There are lots of little jobs the body "does without" when water is scarce. We force it to prioritize. We can get by without these functions for a little while, but eventually the grass will die, we can't see out of the car windows, and the children drive us crazy wanting to get out of the house and do something.

Failure to attend to small problems leads to bigger ones. If you took chemistry in high school, you know that water is required for a vast number of chemical reactions. This is as true in the body as it is in the lab.

In a body made of 70% water, and a brain made of 85% water, dehydration means major stress. Major stress activates the adrenals which begin a series of hormonal maneuvers aimed at holding water in the body. Hormones close off capillaries so that water doesn't pass through to the surrounding tissues. Since water (in lymph) helps carry oxygen and other nutrients in and wastes out, these functions are impaired in a dehydrated individual.

Physical conditions related to dehydration

In his book, *Your Body's Many Cries for Water*[1], Fereydoon Batmanghelidj, M.D., lists more than 15 specific medical conditions he attributes to lack of water. He describes in detail how the body's natural function has been disrupted by dehydration and how it can be restored by good water drinking habits. These conditions include hypertension, asthma, allergies, cardiovascular disease, obesity, gastric ulcers, and many more.

Because dehydration effects every cell individually, dehydration becomes a factor in every disease and condition from cancer to the common cold. In this section, we'll look at some of these conditions in greater depth so you can fully appreciate the significance of water in your personal health program.

The common cold

The common cold is about as common as it gets. This blight seems to hit everyone, frequently, and it can be so hard to get rid of. Dehydration makes it easier to catch a cold and much harder to shake it off. It also makes the aftermath hard to deal with. As your body begins to ration water, mucous membranes are regarded as less important for survival than major organs so they are among the first tissues to be short-changed. These membranes line your sinuses, your throat, your lungs, and your nasal passages and when they dry out, these tissues' defenses are very low; that's why dehydration makes it easy to catch something.

When sinus and lung tissue is dry and irritated, it's also much easier for a secondary infection of bacterial or fungal origin to set in after the viral threat has been overcome. This can prolong your recovery by days or even weeks as you become highly vulnerable to sinus infection or pneumonia. Mucous-producing tissues soothe, cleanse, and defend themselves by producing mucous to flush irritants out—it takes water to make mucous.

Unfortunately, the first thing most people do for a cold is to grab decongestants and anti-histamines which dry that mucous up and create even more irritation and dehydration in those already inflamed tissues. By the way, antibiotics should never be prescribed for colds. Antibiotics have no effect whatsoever on viruses which cause colds. They only work on bacteria, and they actually cause fungal overgrowth. The vast majority of persistent or recurrent sinus and ear infections are actually yeast infections. Antibiotics only make it worse.

Proper hydration is a first-line defense against all infections of the respiratory system—and the digestive system. The entire digestive system is also lined with mucous-producing tissue.

What your liver and kidneys want you to know…

When we don't drink enough water, everything in the body becomes more concentrated—including wastes. The normal functioning of a healthy body produces waste products—toxins—constantly, and these must find their way through the lymphatic fluids (mostly water) and into the blood stream (also mostly water).

Your liver and kidneys have to filter these out of your blood to remove them from your body; but when you are dehydrated, they come down the conveyor belt too fast. Did you ever see the "I Love Lucy" show? How about the episode where Lucy and Ethel had to wrap candies coming down a conveyor belt? It was easy at first, but then the supervisor decided to speed up the conveyor. Lucy and Ethel couldn't keep up, and chaos ensued. Candy went unwrapped and the ladies got fired.

Let's call your kidneys Lucy and Ethel. When you get dehydrated, the wastes come down the conveyor belt, which is your blood stream, closer together than normal—very concentrated. Lucy and Ethel can't pick these things out of your blood stream and wrap them up fast enough, and some of them go on through and stay in circulation for a few more rounds because the girls are no longer performing well under all this stress.

The same thing happens in your liver, and as toxicity builds up in your body, you just don't feel well. Maybe your aches and pains increase, or you get a headache. Maybe you get a stomachache, or intestinal irritation. How about some allergies or a runny nose?

Deficiencies and fatigue

Thirst is not an early warning system. By the time you feel significantly thirsty you are already 2% dehydrated. When you are 2% dehydrated, your energy production falls by 20-30%. That's a lot. How many people struggle with fatigue every day?

It is very difficult, in a dehydrated body, for nutrients such as vitamins, minerals, and oxygen to reach all of the cells that need them. Energy production will be reduced, cell replacement will slow down. Nothing works as it should. The end result here will be nutrient deficiencies in various places in the body and slower healing. Again, you don't feel so good.

Obesity

The rate of obesity in America is high and getting higher. According to information from the National Health and Nutrition Examination Survey and the CDC, 68% of U.S. adults and 47% of U.S. children are overweight or obese, and diabetes and heart disease are major concerns for these individuals. (http://www.cdc.gov/obesity/index.html) Taken together, these three conditions cost citizens and tax payers billions every year in lost wages due to inability to work, health care costs, and other related expenses.

What's striking about this is that when a body is very dehydrated, thirst is often interpreted as hunger. How many of these people are digging their own graves with a fork and spoon when what they really need is a glass of water?

Providentially enough, drinking water is not only one of the keys to awesome health; it's also a major key to shedding unwanted weight. Statistics show that people who drink enough water have much greater success in weight loss efforts. That makes sense doesn't it? Everything that leaves your body does so through one of your normal channels of elimination and all of those are fully dependent on water to keep things flowing.

Toxins are often stored in fat cells, so as unwanted pounds are shed, toxins are released into the blood stream. The body wants to be sure it can handle the load and it won't readily release what it can't efficiently get rid of. The key concept here is that as you flush out toxins (and stop putting so many back in—see chapter 3) you help flush out the fat, too.

Heart disease

In the May 1, 2002, issue of the *American Journal of Epidemiology*, researchers reported on a six-year study in which those who drank more than 5 glasses of water each day were at least 41% less likely to die from a heart attack during the term of the study than participants who drank less than two glasses. I know, it's a study, but it's pretty basic—and totally logical. (http://online.wsj.com/article/SB121485664867016997.html)

Heart attacks in men and women are often, though not always, very different. Men are more likely to have heavy plaqueing and clot formation that causes obstruction in a vessel leading to the heart. Women are more likely to experience difficulties with arterial spasms and rhythm abnormalities. Both are affected by dehydration.

Dehydration causes accelerated heart rate as the heart races to compensate for the reduced blood volume. It makes abnormal rhythms more likely to occur and more difficult to correct.

Dehydration makes all cells more vulnerable to damage—including the cells of the heart and the cells that line the blood vessels. When damage occurs there, clots may form. Clots in vessels lead to strokes and heart attacks for thousands of people every day. Dehydration also contributes to extremes in blood pressure which makes blood vessel damage and clot formation a lot more likely.

As you become dehydrated, your blood volume can decrease making it difficult for your body to push blood into tissues and organs. Blood is mostly water, you know. What do you do with your water hose when the flow isn't strong enough to move the water where you want it to go? You clamp down on that hose to increase the pressure, right? The muscular layer within your blood vessels can do the same thing—it's one way to experience hypertension. Conversely, as you become increasingly dehydrated, your blood volume may fall so low your blood pressure bottoms out. In most all body processes, balance is everything and the same cause can have effects at both ends of the spectrum.

DNA, dehydration, tissue repair, and cancer

You are, in a sense, made primarily of water, protein, and minerals; that's your structure. Every solid thing in your body is non-liquid because of it's protein structure. Proteins have amazing functionality when they are not damaged. Their 3-dimensional structure can bend without breaking and can be twisted into really complicated, but useful, shapes without breaking. The function of a protein is almost entirely dependent on its shape. This is all possible because of the water that helps hold the protein together.

Water holds things together? Strange though it sounds, yes. Attraction and repulsion in hydro physics are the major factors lending protein its amazingly pliable, "fluid" structure. When water is in short supply in the body, or cooked away from a food, the protein structure is damaged and its function may be lost completely.

The genetic code carried in your DNA gives detailed instructions for every aspect of you. Using this blueprint, it is possible to replace or repair any protein in your body. If you are dehydrated, what do you think happens when it's time to copy the DNA protein that tells your body how to replace or repair one of your 100 trillion cells? The odds of correct DNA replication go down which leaves you vulnerable to a mutation. DNA mutations greatly hinder the process of healing a damaged tissue; they can also initiate the development of cancer.

6 Steps to a well-hydrated you

Drinking water sounds like a simple thing to do. But getting enough water of a quality that will bring you good health actually requires not only some information but also some effort on your part. Here are six steps to help you take control of your water intake.

Step one: De-bunk your story

If you don't already have a good water-drinking habit, chances are you do have a list of reasons to explain why you can't achieve this goal. Step one is to look at these and recognize that they are nothing more than stories you've been telling yourself, and some of them may be really good ones. The trick is in telling the truth.

The truth is that something about what you currently drink is comforting, pleasurable, or just familiar to you, and you don't want to leave it. Our habits give us a visceral experience of identity. Drinking coffee or tea, smoking, drinking alcohol, and eating certain foods are strongly associated with some very specific stereotypes which we can readily latch on to as an identity—at least for a few minutes now and then. It's a way to change your state of mind instantly; it's emotional management; a cheap vacation. Indulging in these things is like Hamburger Helper for your psyche. It's just faster and easier than cooking something up from scratch.

It's hard work being unique all the time. It's uncomfortable. It's also harder to blend in and be part of a group without these crutches. Knowing how you use your drinks will help you make choices and substitutions. For example, if you crave the coffee-house atmosphere with a few friends after work there is no need to give it up. Most establishments offer some excellent and interesting herbal teas which are perfectly fine. You can sit with your friends and your warm mug as long as you like—once the conversation is flowing, no one cares what's in your cup, probably not even you!

Any change of habit causes a change in identity, and that may make you or your friends or family uncomfortable. You have to decide what you want. Change is part of life, and it's inevitable. If your friends can't even accept something as simple as a change in what you drink now, how will they accept you, or your absence, with a debilitating illness later?

If you can accept the possibility that change can be good, and if you can see it for the adventure that it is, you will be able to lead the charge and actively shape your destiny. Reassure yourself and your loved ones that while many old habits may pass away, love is eternal. You will always be there for yourself and for them. (And promise them you won't become a rabid evangelist…)

The only alternative to changing your habits is to change nothing at all. If you can't accept where your life is headed "as is," I suspect the truth is that *you* have already changed. All that you need now is to stop fighting it. It's time to make your habits match the you that you've become.

Now that you have your psychological and relational ducks in a row, it's time for…

Step 2. Stop the pop—sugar is not as sweet as you think

If you have acquired the habit of drinking pop and coffee every day, you have to stop it to regain your health. "But drinking a few cans of pop can't be that big a deal, right? It's not like I'm filling a coffee cup with pure table sugar and eating it with a spoon!" Well, actually, if you drink 4 cans of pop in a day, you will be having the same amount of sugar that would fill an 8 ounces coffee cup to the normal drinking level—about 12 tablespoons. That's a quarter pound of sugar—an incredibly unhealthy amount, spoon or no spoon.

- U.S. sugar consumption

According to the United States Department of Agriculture (USDA) the average American consumes between *150 to 170 pounds* of sugar in one year. A hundred years ago, it was only about 5 pounds per person. Many people have already shunned the white granules, so for those who eat little or no sugar there are apparently also some out there who are easily putting away upwards of 250 pounds per year—and many of them are our children.

- Sugar and diabetes

Consuming sugar in vast quantities stresses your sugar-handling system and everybody knows that leads to diabetes. It's one of the fastest growing diseases in human history and unless everybody gets wise in a hurry, by 2050 the majority of Americans will have it. Diabetes takes the life of its victims prematurely and makes what's left of it a lot less enjoyable. Daily injections, pills, the possibility of amputations, heart disease, the loss of eyesight and hearing, and the pain of wounds that will not heal await those who become diabetic and don't reverse it. (Yes, you can almost always reverse it.) Stopping the pop is a great help to avoid diabetes and a great first step on the road to reversing it.

- Sugar and your immune system

If obesity and diabetes don't move you, how do you feel about catching colds and other illnesses—often? Sugar consumption reduces your immune system's ability to attack viruses, bacteria, yeasts, and cancer cells by over 50%. According to Jennifer M. Regan, a NASM certified personal trainer and Cancer Wellness Specialist, "The immune-suppressing effect of sugar starts less than thirty minutes after ingestion and may last for five hours."[10]

If you have donuts for breakfast, a can of pop with lunch, and a nice slice of pie after dinner you've shut your immune system down for the entire day—you are walking across the front lines unarmed and unprotected.

- Sugar and cancer

Guess what loves pop even more than movie-goers? Cancer cells. Unlike normal cells which can use fats, sugars, and even proteins for fuel, cancer cells use only the sugar. If they don't get the sugar supply they need, they die. When you feed cancer cells a rich sugar source like pop, they thank you by multiplying rapidly. You tell them what to do by what you eat and drink.

- Sugar and heart disease

When you drink pop instead of water, your blood vessel linings become dehydrated and vulnerable to damage from the sugar in the pop which acts as an irritant to vessel linings, as does the insulin release it causes. What a recipe for disaster! Sugar is also a huge burden to your pancreas, it's hard on your kidneys, and it sticks to the surface of your red blood cells, reducing their ability to carry oxygen to your body.

Artificial sweeteners actually contribute to obesity and cause a host of other problems, so sugar-free chemical sweetener isn't going to solve the problem either. It's my opinion that nothing could possibly taste so good that I don't care what happens to me after I drink it.

Now that you have good reasons to make the switch to water firmly fixed in your mind, you need to know...

Step 3. How much?

After you stop drinking the wrong things, you need to start drinking good old-fashioned water in the right quantities. There is a limit to how much of anything your body can absorb in an hour. Generally, around six to eight ounces per hour is about all the water you can use, unless you are engaged in vigorous sweaty activities.

To calculate your own individual need for the day, write down your weight in pounds. Divide that number in half and drink that many ounces of water each day. If you weigh 100 pounds, you will need 50 ounces of water daily. If you exercise or are out in the heat, add more. (This equation tops out. If you weigh more than 300 pounds, you can't use it. Don't drink more than 150 ounces of water per day unless you are working hard in the heat.)

Your body prefers that you maintain a steady water supply throughout the day. Don't gulp 25 ounces in the morning and another 25 right before bed. Pace yourself.

Don't be surprised if your body doesn't believe you right away. It's not unusual to feel that you are urinating out all that you're trying to put in for the first couple of days. You will begin to hold on to the water more as you go along.

One sign that you're making progress on re-hydrating your body is the light color of the urine you produce. When it is yellow, orange, or brown, and when it has a strong odor, these may be signs that you are very dehydrated. Although these symptoms will likely pass quickly, it will take more time to fully re-hydrate distant tissues such as your eyes or tissues with limited blood supply such as your joints.

Now that you know how much you need, it's time to:

Step 4. Choose your source

• What's wrong with tap water?

You will need to give some attention to what type of water you drink and where it comes from. Most people are at least mildly displeased with the taste of tap water. If you dislike it, you won't drink it. I don't believe that tap water is high quality water because of what your local water company can't filter out and because of what has been added in.

Since the mid 1900s, U.S. water supplies have been purposefully contaminated with fluoride and chlorine. These elements, along with bromine, are part of the same chemical family in the periodic table. Another brother is iodine. Because fluoride and chlorine are stronger than iodine, they will displace iodine from your body, as will the bromine found in many bread products. Displacing iodine reduces your body's production of thyroid hormone because all thyroid hormones are built on the foundation of iodine. T3 means three iodine are present, T4 has four.

If you suffer from fibromyalgia, chronic fatigue, or any neurological dysfunction, you should seriously consider the role of fluoride in your life.

It is a well-known and potent neurotoxin. The symptoms of overt fluoride poisoning are remarkably similar to the symptoms of fibromyalgia and chronic fatigue.

Few people realize the many ways we are exposed to fluoride. Children are routinely treated with large doses of this neurotoxin twice annually at dentist's offices—any connection to the ADHD epidemic? I don't know. Adults are routinely exposed through antibiotics and other drugs with high levels of fluorides in them. Virtually all of us have been exposed through water, toothpaste, and other oral hygiene products.

Another problem with fluoride is that it's actually bad for your bones. Fluoride in water and toothpaste has been marketed to us as beneficial for our teeth, but it's far from helpful. Naturally occurring fluoride as found in plants is a micronutrient we require in miniscule quantities. The right kind of fluoride, in the right quantity, does help to harden bone and enamel[3].

The toxic waste fluoride that has been routinely added to our toothpaste and dumped into our water supply not only exceeds the human need for fluoride, but it's also in the wrong form. Excessive fluoride is well known to cause brittle teeth and bones. While it does harden the enamel of your teeth, it also makes it thinner. Thin and brittle are not the words I'd like to use to describe the enamel of my teeth. If you look for it, there is an understated warning label on your toothpaste box.

My other objection to tap water is that it is far too contaminated to be healthy. Here are three sources of contaminants that flow from your faucet every day:

1. Asbestos is in the water supply because many years ago, when no one knew better, hundreds of thousands of miles of concrete conduit were laid underground to carry water to our households. This concrete contained asbestos. The current EPA protective standard allows 7 million, yes million, asbestos fibers per liter of tap water.[3] I don't want to drink that.

2. It's really hard to top the asbestos, but keep in mind that Americans, per capita, are taking more medications than ever before in human history. These antibiotics, chemotherapy drugs, anti-psychotic drugs, and synthetic hormones are metabolized by the body and eliminated. They end up in the water supply and municipal treatment facilities were never designed to remove them all.

3. I drove down my own street yesterday and saw a huge truck spraying hundreds of gallons of heavy-duty herbicide over a neighbor's field. He's preparing to plant this year's crop of GMO corn, so he's using

more pesticide and herbicide than ever. It all runs into our water supply.

For those who are dedicated to their health, tap water just won't get the job done. Our goal is to raise standards, so consider these alternatives to the tap.

• Distilled water. Some people advocate strongly for or against distilled water. I personally believe it is a very good alternative. If you like, you can purchase a distiller for your home inexpensively to save money in the long run on buying water. Be aware that if you buy distilled water in the store, at least some states allow bottlers to use a percentage of tap water in their distilled water jugs.

I don't think it is a problem, but if the lack of minerals in distilled water concerns you, add some trace mineral drops (Concentrace or Watermax are two good brands) to your distilled water. Distilled water is the surest way to be certain you have a very clean source of healthy water. I have a distiller, and I drink distilled water. I keep it in a large glass dispenser to avoid plastic leaching into it.

• Purified water you bottle yourself. There are many stores now offering a water purification machine for public use. Many locations of Walmart, many health food stores, and some grocery stores offer this for a very small fee per gallon. You bring your own jug and fill it yourself. This is a cost-effective method for getting water of reliable quality. The system uses multiple mechanisms for removing objectionable contaminants from existing city water. I buy this water to use for cooking.

• Spring water. The quality of bottled spring water varies tremendously. In some cases it is high quality, but I wouldn't buy it unless there was detailed information about its quality listed on the bottle. Even then, there are no guarantees. There is uncertainty about the regulation of the industry because so many spring waters are bottled in other countries. Spring water has the potential to be some of the best water or some of the worst; the risk of contamination is real.

• Drinking water. Water labeled "drinking water" is often nothing more than city tap water. If you look at the back of the bottle it will usually say that it was obtained from a "municipal source." That means tap water. It's cheap, but it's still a huge rip off.

Whatever you choose, never leave plastic bottles in a hot car. Chemicals leach out of the plastic into the water. Some of these chemicals have a disruptive effect on your hormonal balance, and all chemicals are toxic to your liver.

Now that you have some good water, you still have one issue...

Step 5. Taste matters

It is a reality that some people just don't like water, and that makes it hard for them to drink it without feeling really deprived. While water may not be exciting or glamorous, it is another example of something elegantly simple that we can learn to appreciate even if we don't greatly enjoy it. Water can do us a tremendous amount of good if we will only use it to its full advantage.

Remember, attitude is everything. If you believe the Bible, then you believe that the first humans were created and placed in a garden with all they needed for abundant living. I believe that's true, but I also know that abundant living takes us back to those attitude and perception issues we talked about in chapter 1. Let's look at it from the standpoint of what Adam and Eve didn't have for a moment: no house, no car, no income, and no clothes! No Walmart, no Kroger, no internet, and no doctor.

If you're a glass-half-full person, you could also say: no mortgage, no high gas prices, no annoying boss, and no laundry! No long check-out lines, no choosing paper or plastic, no slow downloads, and no health insurance crisis. Perspective management allows us to be grateful for good clean water, and gratitude enables us to be happy while we drink it—even if we don't like it.

If you are accustomed to strong tastes, it may be difficult for you to make a change, but don't despair, there are ways to add flavor without adding chemicals or sugars. No pop, no coffee, and no black tea doesn't have to mean no sweetness, no taste, and no fun.

An herbal product called stevia adds tremendous sweetness, and it comes in a variety of flavors as well. Most health food stores and some groceries carry this product in liquid or powdered forms. It has no calories, no chemicals, and no harmful side effects. It is safe for all ages and conditions—including diabetes. There is no harm in adding a drop or two to a bottle of water to add some flavor if it will get you into the habit of drinking your water. This works well for children who are addicted to too much pasteurized fruit juice.

Another way to handle the taste issue is to squeeze some fresh lemon or lime juice into your water. Some people also enjoy the mild taste of sliced berries or a few sprigs of mint leaf left to float in a pitcher of water for a few hours. Once removed, the leaves or berries leave a lingering essence in the water. Try raspberries, blueberries, strawberries, or blackberries. You might just go from envying your friends' pop, to having your friends envying what's in your bottle.

Adding herbal teas to the water can be a nice change as well. Avoid the black teas and stick strictly with herbs to avoid the dehydrating effects and caffeine that black teas contribute. Chamomile is nice and relaxing, elderberry and rose hips are strengthening to the immune system, and licorice root is extremely sweet and very good for the stomach and the adrenal glands—but don't use it all the time as it may have some potential for elevating blood pressure.

There are dozens of interesting choices and many health food stores now offer herbs in bulk—you just scoop out as much as you like from a large jar. It is extremely economical. Ask your local health food store for advice or a quick tour of their bulk section.

You've got all the physical elements in place. Now it's time to:

Step 6. Make your plan

There are several ways to cultivate good habits; planning is always an important part of the process. Consider what sort of container you will use. It needs to suit your taste and your lifestyle. If you are fortunate enough to work in a building where a water cooler is provided, all you need is your favorite coffee cup and you're all set. If you need to carry your water with you, you may like to take a gallon jug to work and get your refills from that.

If you don't work but are in the car a lot running errands or chauffeuring children, you may like to take one or more purse-appropriate, or car-appropriate, water bottles pre-filled and re-load your bag when one is empty. I prefer glass or stainless steel bottles instead of plastic to be sure my water isn't full of chemicals, especially in a hot car. The important point is, one way or another, don't leave home without your water, or at least not without knowing where you'll get it.

Think through how you will drink throughout the day. Will you set up an hourly chime on your watch or computer to remind yourself? Will you aim for eight ounces per hour, four ounces per half hour? When will you start and when will you finish? Allowing a couple of water-free hours before bedtime is always a good idea, lest you be awakened to get up and go in the night.

Here's what works for me. I know I need about 60 ounces of high-quality liquid every day. I know that I will be drinking 12 to 16 ounces of fresh vegetable juice, so that leaves me with a water requirement of around 48 ounces. I keep 2 inexpensive stainless steel bottles that each hold 24 ounces. Every morning, I rinse them out and refill them from my distiller. I drink one between 8:00 a.m. and 2:00 p.m., another between 2:00 p.m. and 8:00 p.m. When I leave the house, they go with me. One stays in my bag, the other in the car until it's time to switch them. This is what works for me.

Having a buddy to go through this program with is always a great idea. If you have a friend who would be interested in doing this together, that makes it a lot more fun and increases your chances of success tremendously. You can remind each other, encourage each other, and challenge each other to achieve your goals. You don't have to have identical standards or goals, just a similar drive to succeed and a genuine desire to help each other reach your different goals.

What exactly did God provide for the health of His human creations? He gave us abundant fresh produce ready to pick, fresh air, fair weather, and lots of good clean water. I admit there is a good chance that I wasn't the first to think of the 7 Keys… Good health was always part of the plan; we've just forgotten how to execute it. Acquiring good drinking habits is the second milestone on your journey. I challenge you to take the following six steps to master this second key to awesome health.

Review

Key #2 Water

Hydration recovery plan

Step one: De-bunk your story / identify your psychological needs.

Step two: Stop the pop.

Step three: Figure out how much you need every day.

Step four: Choose your source.

Step five: Make it taste good.

Step six: Plan for success.

Chapter 3: Elimination

In a sense this chapter is all about stress. There are many kinds or sources of stress, but they all have one thing in common—they're hard on your mind and your body. While some attempt to categorize stressful events as positive or negative, it may be more productive to recognize that it is the quantity and intensity of events that decides whether the stress will be positive or negative for you at any given moment.

Some events, such as the death of a loved one, automatically cross the line due to intensity. Other events, such as a job change, may be positive or negative depending on how much other stress you were already dealing with when it happened.

The 7 Keys to AWESOME health described in this book have three things in common:

1. They can be sources of additional stress if you don't take control of them.

2. They can be the keys to your healing if you do take charge and manage them correctly.

3. They are all within your control right now.

Clean your house

As you begin the mission of reclaiming your health, there are some things that just need to go. When you do a major house-cleaning, you probably begin by looking around and spotting a few things that have been hanging around for years cluttering up your place. These things are broken, unattractive, or out of date. There isn't a better place for them and they can't be fixed. It's just time to get rid of them.

Unlike broken appliances and pictures of dogs playing poker, bad habits usually do serve some purpose in our lives. Review chapter one. It may not be a good purpose, but if you drop a bad habit cold turkey, you will suffer and you may relapse quickly. While failure is one oft-repeated step on the rocky road of success, it isn't fun and we all want to prevent it.

The trick is to identify what purpose a bad habit serves for you and plan how you will address that need without the bad habit. A good plan usually consists of healthier substitutions, appropriate emotional support, and real clarity about why you want to do this

There are several categories of things you may need to greatly reduce or, preferably, eliminate from your life if you truly want to master your health. To be specific there are dangerous substances you can eat, drink, inhale, or inject; dangerous things you can view or listen to; and dangerous relationships you could be involved in. Elimination is truly one of the most difficult steps to implement.

While there is merit in the idea of moderation, that concept applies only to things that actually have at least some merit. Some things just aren't good for you in any quantity. Rat poison, for example, is something you just don't need—not even a little bit. That's a very black and white issue—it's easy to understand that every single bite is harmful. Unfortunately, most of us are conditioned to see other unhealthy ideas in various shades of gray even though every exposure, even a little one, truly is harmful.

Substance abuse is, of course, the most serious of the habits you must eliminate for the sake of your health. There are millions of printed pages dedicated to graphic descriptions of the horrors that await those who become involved with illegal (and even legal) drugs; smoking; and alcohol. Most people reading a book like this one have already rejected those paths, so let's just leave it at: never, never, and never.

There are other substances even the most upstanding people have yet to reject which, none the less, wreak havoc on the population—costing us billions in healthcare dollars each year and leaving a trail of suffering victims, grieving families, and unanswered questions in their wake. When I name them, you may doubt that these "harmless" common substances could ever be responsible for so much heartache, but it's entirely true.

Step 1. 4F failing foods

There are four categories of edibles (I hesitate to call them foods) that you need to eliminate if you want to be well. Eliminating these is Step 1 in your effort to eliminate what's hurting you. In military terms, a designation of 4F means that you are unfit for service because you don't meet the minimum standards established. The following foods are 4F— they are unfit for service. They all begin with the letter "F," and they get an "F" for their total failure to meet the nutritional needs of the American population.

1. Fried foods (prepared by cooking in a pot of hot oil)
2. Fragmented and fortified foods (having nutrients purposefully removed by the manufacturer and/or having low-quality synthetic vitamins added during processing)
3. Foods with a face (animal products)
4. Franken-foods (genetically altered products)

I know; there isn't anything left in America to eat. What about our cultural need for fast food? It starts with an F, too, because most fast food breaks ALL 4 rules above—even fast-food salads often break these rules. If you feel like you just fell off your horse, any decent trainer would tell you to get right back on. Don't stop reading now.

These 4 Fs contain the vast majority of dietary toxins people consume. Weight control is closely related to toxicity and inflammation. There are some diets that promise weight loss while you continue eating the same 4F foods that brought you here. These diets will never allow you to rid your body of toxins and inflammation—which cause disease. The only way to lose weight and recover your health is to detoxify your body. As the toxins go, excess weight will go too. It's no use looking fit and trim at your own funeral.

Hopefully if you had a "friend" who beat the daylights out of you every time he came to your house you'd stop asking him over. The four categories of foods mentioned above are literally beating the daylights out of people all over the world who have adopted the Standard American Diet. (SAD) If our government outlawed the four categories above, and did nothing else, our world would change dramatically in less than one year.

I want to coin a new medical term: Standard American Diet Syndrome. That's what we could rightly say is behind so many of the symptoms we see people experiencing everywhere. Cardiovascular disease, diabetes, cancer, digestive disorders, low immunity—all of these are really one disease. Standard American Diet Syndrome.

Don't believe me? Consider these facts: The enlightening documentary, *Forks Over Knives,* presents the following statistics from the World War II era. Prior to 1940, the death rate from heart attacks and strokes in Norway was rising rapidly. Then something happened that turned the trend upside down fast. When the Germans invaded Norway, they confiscated all the farm animals to feed their own soldiers. The Norwegians were forced, quite suddenly, to adopt a plant-based diet. The result was that the death rate from cardiovascular causes took a sudden dive. What happened when the Germans left? The trend reversed again, and by 1948, the death rate was back up near the 1940 level.

If we all got rid of the 4F foods, thousands of people would begin to recover from heart disease, many cancers would stop forming and growing, chemical production and usage would drop, and the incidence of diabetes especially among children would drop dramatically. There would be only a fraction of the hospital admissions, a fraction of the work days lost to illness, you get the idea. Why are these foods so bad?

The simple answer is that the human body wasn't made to handle them. Why can't your car run on yogurt? It wasn't made that way! Our modern dietary habits are the physiological equivalent of pouring sand into the gas tank of an old Tin Lizzie and expecting to win the Indy 500. It's amazing we do so well.

Fried foods

Fried food is a problem because of what deep frying does to fats. Hydrogenation is a process that spontaneously occurs in fats at very high heat. It is also done purposefully in factories. Hydrogenation adds extra hydrogen to the chemical structure of the fat which makes it remain solid at room temperature. This is how we get products like margarine and shortening. I think shortening is an exceptionally well-chosen name for the product because it will very likely shorten your lifespan if you continue to eat it in any quantity.

Sometimes the hydrogenation is only partial, but it is still just as dangerous, perhaps even more so as it is the partial hydrogenation which is responsible for creating the infamous trans-fats. The human body can not use hydrogenated fats, which really are damaged fats, to build healthy cells. It's like trying to repair your car with broken parts.

You must build millions of new cells every day to replace those that die. Each cell has a membrane surrounding it that separates it from its immediate environment and determines what can pass into and out of the cell itself. Fat molecules are major components in the membrane of every cell. If you build the membranes of your cells with damaged fats, your cell membranes won't function properly. Things will get in that shouldn't; things won't get out that should.

When membranes don't function properly, your cells' defenses will be greatly compromised, and bacteria and viruses will find you easy prey. With poor defenses, cell damage is far more likely, and the end result of cell damage that can't be successfully repaired is either cell death or cancer. With a poor diet, you don't have what you need to repair the damage.

Fragmented (refined) and fortified foods

Fragmented foods and fortified foods are usually one and the same—and logically so. Another name for fragmented food is "refined" food. "Refined" sounds nice. A refined person is someone who has removed from his or her personality many little habits or mannerisms that might cause annoyance or offence to others. But what about a refined food? What did they take out?

The brown stuff they take out of flour is the bran and the germ. The bran contains good whole B vitamins in their natural context, while the germ contains the whole vitamin E complex. The white part left behind is starch. Starch is nothing but a form of sugar—with practically no nutrients at all. Why would they do that?

A while back, people figured out how to make flour and sugar whiter and fluffier. When you take out the wheat bran and the wheat germ, the flour makes fluffier cakes and light airy breads that people really enjoy. White sugar pours easier than brown. Bugs don't like white flour nearly as well as brown, and white (refined) things keep longer on the shelves. Bleach makes things whiter still, and people like the idea that they are buying something "pure."

Still, some complained about vitamins and minerals being removed from our food supply. After all, deficiency diseases are real. So they created "fortified" or "enriched" foods to make us feel better about what we were eating.

"Fortified" sounds really good; so does "enriched." They've added vitamins and minerals; what's wrong with that? All fortified foods started out as fragmented foods. Imagine you are walking through Central Park one evening. Suddenly, a man approaches. He has a gun, so you follow his instructions and hand over all your valuables. Instead of simply running away to squander your hard-earned money like most robbers, this one has a perverse sense of humor. After taking all your money, your jewelry, and your cell phone, he cackles fiendishly, "I'm going to make you rich tonight." Next, he hands you a quarter and tells you to go call someone and tell them how rich you are. Now you know what it feels like to be "enriched" or "fortified." It feels like adding insult to injury.

In my opinion, when you take away fifty naturally occurring nutrients and add back 3 fake ones, you have no right to say you've fortified anything. Unlike highly perishable naturally occurring vitamins, chemicals last a long, long time. That very difference should tell you synthetic vitamins aren't the same as real ones. They might satisfy the government definition for a vitamin, but they operate radically differently in your body, just as they do in the bag on the shelf. Your body was not made to run on factory chemicals. These "fake" vitamins are ultimately regarded by your body as toxins—more garbage to take out.

Food with a face

This one is the breaking point for many people, especially men. There is so much cultural mythology built up around the concept of eating animals. It's very "manly" in our culture to consume large amounts of meat. Many people feel you aren't a "real man" if you don't put away a half-pound or so of porterhouse in public.

Apart from gender issues, many more people are very misinformed about the nutritional "necessity" of meat. Most Americans are absolutely convinced that you can not expect to be strong or live long without meat; that you need large amounts of protein; and that you will become vitamin and mineral deficient without lots of meat in your diet. Rather than asking, "Where's the beef," we should be asking, "Where's the truth?"

There was a time when government recommendations suggested that meat was necessary for health. Most people don't realize that in more recent decades, the government recommendations have been significantly changed to reflect more accurate data. The USDA now clearly states that being vegetarian is a healthy option.[11] They also clearly recognize the important role of fruits and vegetables in human health and they consistently recommend more and more of them in each new iteration of dietary guidelines. My complaint with the USDA is that I don't believe they have yet caught up with current research or logic—they don't go nearly far enough.

The case against meat

Consider several facts about meat:

1. In order to safely ingest and digest meat, a creature needs stomach acid much stronger than anything a human is capable of manufacturing. Your dog can safely eat raw meat and eggs; the health risk warning on the carton is for you.

2. Herbivores digest mainly in the intestinal tract. They need long, narrow, winding intestines to help them slowly extract the nutrients from the fiber in their diet. Carnivores digest food more rapidly—about 8 hours compared with our 24. They need short, wide, fairly straight intestines to rapidly pass the remains of their diet before it begins to decompose. Guess which kind you have? (Hint: You are not a carnivore.)

3. True carnivores have NO flat, grinding molars. How many do you have?

4. The canine teeth of a carnivore are large and effective for tearing raw flesh. Yours are puny by comparison and not at all effective at tearing raw flesh. Want to try it?

5. The largest animals in the world need more protein and calories than you do, and they eat grasses and grains, not meat.

6. The animals you get your protein from got theirs from eating plants. (Nobody eats carnivores. I've heard cannibals don't even like to eat Americans.)

7. People who try extreme diets consisting almost entirely of animal products eventually become very ill. People who try diets consisting almost exclusively of fresh fruits and vegetables become healthier.

8. The average life span for plant-eating animals is much longer than for meat-eating animals.

9. A human baby's need for protein for growth far exceeds the need of an adult, yet the perfect food for human babies, human milk, is not more than 5% protein. How much do you really need?

10. There is protein in every fruit, every vegetable, every nut, and every seed. In some vegetables, and most nuts, there is more protein per 100 calories than in meat.

11. Protein in meat and dairy products has been found to stimulate growth of cancer cells. Protein in plants has been found not to.

12. Many Olympians and other highly successful professional athletes are strict vegetarians. They have lots of energy, strong bones and muscles, and numerous medals. Here's a short list of vegetarian athletes:

   . Henry Aaron, all-time major league home run champion
   . Ridgely Abele, eight national championships in karate
   . Andreas Cahling, Mr. International body building champion
   . Estelle Gray and Cheryl Marek, world record in cross-country tandem cycling
   . Roy Hilligan, Mr. America body building champion
   . Sixto Linares, world record holder in the 24-hour triathlon
   . Dan Millman, world champion gymnast
   . Paavo Nurmi, 20 world records and nine Olympic medals in distance running

- Stan Price, world record holder in the bench press
- Murray Rose, world records in the 400 and 1500-meter freestyle
- Dave Scott, six-time winner of the Ironman Triathlon (the only man to win it more than twice!)

Please understand, I am not suggesting that your health hangs fully in the balance over your decision to eat meat tonight. There are a lot of factors; seven that I can think of immediately. I would hate to see a couple arguing over his steak while she's binging on an oversized slice of cheesecake. My point is that both are bad, even though neither will kill you outright on a case-by-case basis. Neither is something you want to make a habit of because both are detrimental to your health.

How could meat be bad for you? The same way sand is bad in your gas tank, meat is bad in your gut —you weren't made to handle it. I feed my dogs raw meat, and they are healthy. I don't feed that to my children. Dog food for dogs, people food for people, plant food for plants. Anything you can't handle correctly becomes a poison to you, even if some other creature can thrive on it. This isn't about your dog or the lions at the zoo; it's about you.

Speaking of lions, during the early 1900s, zookeepers, in an honest attempt to keep their big cats fed on a tight budget, started giving them cooked meat left-overs from local restaurants. They quickly became ill, not from eating meat, but from eating it cooked. A study of this phenomenon at the Philadelphia Zoo was described in 1923 by Dr. H. Fox in a book titled *Disease in Captive Wild Animals and Birds*[14]. What nutrition can be gained from meat is partially ruined when you cook it.

When you buy a new pet, a type you've never had before, what's the first question you ask the shop keeper or the vet? "What do I feed it?" Why do we ask that? Because we know, intuitively, that different species eat different things because they have different needs. We know that feeding them the wrong kind of food can kill them or make them sick. Why don't we realize we're the same? Not all food is people food. There is no gastric magic that will transform whatever you swallow into something that will nourish your body.

Most people eating cheesecake are aware, at least on some level, that they are making a less than stellar choice, but I want you to realize that the steak is not better for you. Both are unnecessary and unhealthy indulgences that do nothing to enhance your health. Both cause measurable harm—even in "moderation."

You should not delude yourself with the notion that there is good calcium in the cheesecake that will in any way offset the damage the gross amounts of sugar and bad fat will cause. Neither should you fancy that there is some magical nutritional golden nugget hidden in the grisly depths of hot, dead animal flesh that will redeem you from the ill effect caused by the denatured animal protein load with which you are burdening your body and challenging your pH.

You also should not think that one type of meat is better than another with the possible, barely admissible exception that oily fish may have some redeeming quality over the rest—but it still causes harm. Chicken, beef, pork, and fish are all meats, and all exert similar ill effects on the bodies of those who eat them. There is no benefit you can receive from meat of any kind that you are not better equipped to obtain from plant sources or high-quality whole food supplements.

What harm does meat do?

What is this harm? Why would it be better to get your protein, and your other nutrients, from a plant? It's a simple matter of design and function. That long, winding digestive tract of yours is so well-suited to the slow extraction of nutrients from fiber. It has the absorptive surface area of a football field—literally. It is very convoluted with little hair-like projections everywhere, called villi, that take in nutrients. Even these little hairs are covered with more, tinier nutrient-grabbing hairs—microvilli.

It's easy to see how thick, fiberless substances like meat would gum up these works. Because it has no fiber, and because of the shear length and diameter of your intestine, meat can't pass through your digestive tract quickly enough to prevent it from rotting. Humans have, optimally, a transit time of nearly 24 hours. That means 24 hours from the time you swallow a food to the time you excrete the waste. 24 hours in a warm moist environment will cause meat to rot and it may be much longer because meat can slow your transit time substantially. That rot introduces all sorts of toxic substances into your bloodstream, and it damages the lining of your digestive tract. There's just no way around it.

Chemical, hormonal, and bacterial dangers associated with meat

Another beef I have with the meat industry, is that they absolutely refuse to be responsible with regard to their use of chemicals. If you want to reduce your total intake of harmful pesticides, antibiotics, and synthetic hormones, you need to realize that meat is the richest source for all of those. Toxins are concentrated in the flesh of animals who eat them.

I raise horses and goats, so I'm a frequent customer at the feed stores. I can tell you, it's just about impossible to buy feed for cows without antibiotics already in it. They don't put that in there to keep the cows healthy. They put antibiotics in cow feed because it makes them gain weight faster—unhealthy, unnatural weight. I don't want to eat that.

Chickens are fed synthetic hormones to increase their size, especially the size of the breast. Is that something you need in your diet? How about your daughter? Don't forget that estrogen dominance is strongly correlated with breast cancer.

The final problem I want to mention with regard to the meat industry is the filth of it. According to a safety analysis published on April 15, 2011, in the journal *Clinical Infectious Diseases*[15], 47% of meat and poultry samples taken from U.S. grocery stores were contaminated with staph aureus bacteria. And 52% of the contaminated samples were resistant to three or more classes of antibiotics. That means about 25% of all U.S. meat and poultry is contaminated with antibiotic-resistant bacteria which can cause severe illness or death. S. aureus is the same species we now know as MRSA. It causes a wide range of illnesses from minor skin infections to life-threatening diseases, such as pneumonia, endocarditis, and sepsis. I don't even want this stuff in my house, never mind in my body!

I always have someone who asks about hunting. Fresh game doesn't have all that contamination so it's better, right? Yes, it's better. If you are determined to have a piece of meat, that's clearly the best way to have it.

If you must indulge...

Logically you must know that there is no mineral or vitamin in cow, pig, or fish flesh that did not originate in the plant kingdom. There are no original vitamins or minerals in any animal—that's why animals need to eat in the first place. Plants make their own food; you can't, and neither can the cow, pig, or fish. We think we need milk for calcium, yet we never consider where the cow got it.

Cows don't make calcium, they eat calcium—and you can, too. There is no reason to think that a meatless diet means vitamin or mineral deficiency. If it did, then the animal you want to eat would also be deficient due to his plant-based diet, and he would have nothing to offer you.

Eggs and dairy products present similar problems. When dairy is pasteurized, the enzymes in it are destroyed, the proteins are altered, and the balance of flora is skewed. Commercially produced eggs aren't safe to eat raw anymore, and even if they were, it's important to remember that eggs were designed to feed baby chickens and cow milk was designed for baby cows—not for humans.

I do think that there is less harm in free-range organic eggs, non-pasteurized organic goat milk, organic butter, and raw organic cheeses than in their less natural counterparts, non-organic, caged, grain-fed, and pasteurized. Like meat, these are fiberless substances that can slow transit time, but they do have their enzymes intact.

If you must indulge, these are the best ways to do so, but if you are fighting disease, these indulgences are *not* for you. Even if you're basically healthy, don't think that because I say these are less harmful you can eat all you want of them and maintain perfect health. You can't. You still weren't designed to eat these things in any significant quantity—they are indulgences which have to be paid for. The price is lots and lots of fresh, healthy vegetables to offset them.

Two camps in the field of natural health

There are two basic camps in the nutrition field, and animal products are the focal point of their differences. If you find someone who supports meat-eating, you'll probably find that they take their stand based, if you trace it back far enough, on the work of Weston Price, Sally Fallon, and Mary Enig. Fallon and Enig rely somewhat on Price to back up their arguments for meat consumption. Some meat enthusiasts also owe their stance to government efforts to spread pro-meat and dairy sentiment to bolster sales in those industries.

It's important to realize that Weston Price was *not* attempting to study animal-based versus plant-based diets. Weston Price studied, primarily, the effect of food refining and the introduction of adulterated, chemically-saturated foods into the diets of native populations. He wrote his book *Nutrition and Physical Degeneration* in 1939. We've learned a lot since then, but his actual premise is very true: refined foods and chemicals bring rapid degenerative changes to every population into which they are introduced.

I want to point out that while I disagree with Fallon and Enig on the value of animal products, we do all agree on the importance of fresh fruits and veggies. Both Fallon and Enig have done some good work in nutrition—such as Enig's efforts to alert the world to the dangers of trans-fats.

T. Colin Campbell, on the other hand, *did* study plant-based versus animal-based diets. He concluded that plant-based diets are superior to animal-based diets in human nutrition. Campbell's work showed that animal proteins stimulated cancer growth while plant proteins did not.

Caldwell Esselstyn and Dean Ornish have done excellent work with cardiovascular patients to reverse severe heart disease. Both of them insist that their patients adhere to strict vegan diets and their successes are well-documented. Their patients are still alive and you could probably ask them yourself what diet caused and what diet cured their conditions.

I have yet to see a single clinic anywhere specializing in the reversal of heart disease using an animal-based, protein- and fat-heavy diet. Many people are writing very short books suggesting that animal-based diets are unfairly labeled as being harmful for your heart, but I see no proof. I tried to look one of them up recently and found that the author had already died suddenly of a stroke. He was still in his forties.

Are there people who eat lots of meat and remain healthy? Yes. There are also chain smokers who manage to live a long functional life against the odds, but that doesn't mean we should all light up for health!

How do people eat meat and stay healthy? They back up their meaty diets with a lot of really fine vegetables, fruits, and whole grains. They don't fry everything. They eliminate refined sugars. They frequently take a lot of vitamins, and some of the more well-informed take a lot of acid-forming supplements and enzymes to help them digest their meat. They know their system can't handle it without help, and neither can yours. They won't remain disease-free forever, either.

Yeah, but you know somebody who… Well, all I can tell you is keep watching. The human body is very well-engineered to take a lot of abuse without breaking down, but those back-ups and compensations can't save you forever. Eventually you wear out your back-up systems, you can't compensate for your bad habits any longer, and disease sets in hard and fast. Good nutrition is about prolonging optimal function so you aren't living on back-ups and compensations.

It has been hard for me to write this chapter. Not because I don't know what to say, but because I don't know how to say it so everyone will be okay with it. I don't think that's possible.

Many who hold the view that people were meant to eat meat base their arguments on the principles of the theory of evolution—some don't realize that's where their arguments come from. If you don't believe in evolution, how can you believe in nutritional theories based on evolution?

I was not a tree-hugging, bunny-saving activist when I began to study health and nutrition. In fact I was personally fattening two Holstein calves in my barn in eager anticipation. My grandmother made the best pot roast on earth, and I enjoyed it, a lot. My mother made the best beef brisket you could ever dream of, and I ate a lot of it. I didn't want to give up my meat, but I did it because I learned why it wasn't serving my body or my purpose very well.

So I've studied both sides, honestly. I've listened to brilliant men and women in seminars who swear that human kind were meant from the moment they first crawled out of the ooze to spend every waking minute hunting down and polishing off the bones of less fortunate animals. I appreciate their logic; I appreciate their time and their dedication. I respect their right to hold that opinion, and I ask them to respect mine. We will never all agree on this.

Decide for yourself

Eventually you get to the point where you have to decide for yourself. As I said, I have had many teachers from both sides of the vegetarian fence. Some advocated strongly and logically for meat. Some advocated equally well for vegetables. I remained undecided for some time while I evaluated things and tried to figure out a reliable method for determining what was best.

It soon became apparent that I would never find "the" definitive scientific study that would settle the question once and for all. The contradictions were endless and the money maze impossible to fully trace. Here are the factors that eventually stood out to help me identify the truth:

1. Even though some of my teachers advocated for a lot of animal products in the human diet, not one of them suggested that anyone could be healthy for very long without ALSO eating a lot of high-quality vegetables. I began to see that that was where all the nutrition was really coming from.

2. I grew up eating plenty of meat and I felt terrible. I switched to a plant-based diet and I improved dramatically. More than ten years later, I'm still going strong.

3. Within a five-year period, 75% of my teachers who advocated an animal-based diet were dead. Not one of them died of old age.

4. 100% of my teachers who advocated a plant-based diet are still alive and thriving. None of them look their age.

5. In Genesis 1:29, God implemented a plant-based diet for mankind. Meat was not *allowed*, and certainly not commanded, until hundreds of years later, as described in chapter 9. (Faith and gratitude are commanded in the New Testament, but meat consumption is not.)

You will never agree with everyone on diet principles either; the camp will forever remain divided. I've tried it both ways and I suggest that, in the interest of real science, you do the same before you make a decision. It has to be an honest attempt—a week isn't going to do it. Changing your diet half-way won't do it. Changing diet without addressing the other six keys won't do it either.

Three to six months of full-scale effort on all 7 Keys is required before you have any grounds to say this won't work. Even if you decide this "isn't for you," have the decency to respect others' right to see for themselves. I have not chosen to use my book to bash anybody else's opinions, so I would appreciate the same consideration.

Franken-foods

I find it morally reprehensible that our government, in contrast to other governments in the industrialized world, refuses to allow us the basic human right of knowing and choosing what we are eating. It is vitally important that you realize that government is far more interested in protecting industry than individuals. You and I are sacrificed on the altar of the American economy daily. Genetically modified foods, like many chemical additives, are not at all proven to be safe, and they are already practically everywhere. There is growing evidence that genetically modified foods damage the organs of those who eat them.

These crops do not in any way represent a boon to mankind or relief from world hunger. Quite the opposite, they are absolutely nothing more than the twisted efforts of a few greedy chemists to dominate the world at one of its most vulnerable points—the food supply. We really need to wake up and start demanding our rights before we all have a "body by <chemical company> label" tattooed across our backsides.

Forgetting for a moment that we have no idea what ill effect eating these modified foods will have on our bodies long-term, we need to be aware of some short-term consequences that may be dire. When genes from one plant are added to another, people who are allergic to the one may also react to the other. This effect has already been documented. These anaphylactic reactions are life-threatening. Not only are we not told a product has these specific allergens, we're not even told it contains GMO ingredients.

How can people with food allergies ever be safe? There is no label to tell you what genes are in the food you're eating. If you don't have food allergies, don't feel safe yet. As more foods have more foreign genes, more people will begin to have more allergic reactions, this has already been documented with GMO soy.

How widespread is the GMO problem in our country? Because some of the most common ingredients are now genetically modified, approximately 80% of the non-organic processed foods in the United States now contain GMOs. Even foods labeled "natural" or "all natural" may contain GMOs.

Consider the prevalence of GMO among some of our common crops based on these statistics from www.labelityourself.org:

Canola	90%	Corn	88%
Cotton	94%	Sugar beets	95%

If you continue to eat animal products, be aware that the vast majority of American animals are raised on GMOs. I have personally spoken with the Purina company and they have confirmed that their animal feeds do contain GMOs. I told them I would not be buying feed from them in the future unless their policy was changed. Everything the animals are fed eventually feeds the people who eat animal products.

If you want to learn more about this topic, read the excellent book by Jeffrey M. Smith, *Seeds of Deception*.[9] GMO grain products are in almost every processed, packaged food that does not specifically claim to be GMO free. The only way to protect yourself is to avoid processed food.

A word about genes

My purpose is for everyone to understand their own physiology and make informed decisions. I also want people to understand why they are having health problems. Too many people assume that their disease was genetically programmed into them from the beginning of time and that they have no control over it. The tragic consequence of this errant assumption is a lifetime of disease-management when disease elimination would have been a far more profitable use of a precious lifetime.

While there are tragic chromosomal abnormalities we can't control, most people are afflicted not with problems of genetic abnormality, but with problems of genetic expression.

The truth is that, for most of us, while our genes may determine where our weakest link is, our habits are the bolt cutters that actually sever that link. We all have genetic weaknesses, and therefore we are all capable of producing diseased states; whether we ever express that genetic potential and experience disease is usually up to us. The vast majority of Americans really are digging their own graves one spoonful at a time.

Now that you know what to avoid, it's time to raise your standards. You need to formulate:

An action plan

1. Keep a journal of what you commonly eat every day for at least a week. Write down your new standards for food. Sit down with your journal at the end of the week and circle all the things that don't meet your new standards.

2. Observe your emotions around eating these unhealthy foods. Is it a matter of convenience or of comfort? Is it a social thing or just because you didn't know a better way? Review chapter one to help address psychology issues around this subject.

3. Begin to look for where bad ingredients pop up. Become a label reader and learn what foods tend to have problem ingredients. Remember: the best foods don't even have an ingredient label.

4. Begin to look for alternatives to the things you've decided to avoid while you are at restaurants, at the grocery store, and at home.

5. Take a shopping tour of the local health food store or the health food section of the grocery store, and make a list of ways to substitute healthier options for what you need to get rid of. Think simple at first, don't try to go gourmet too quickly. I would recommend taking a little time just to observe your own emotions around eating bad food. Use the time to finish this book because there will be substantial help for this process in chapter 6 on Maximize Your Nutrition.

6. Get some good cookbooks. There are recipe books out there for raw foods, vegetarian dishes, whatever you need. I'm writing one myself. It's a good idea to get a couple and try some new things. It's also good to skim through some of these to get an overall high-level idea of what sort of ingredient combinations are typical in the style of food prep you've chosen to study. This is a good way to educate yourself on how to stock your pantry. You'll be able to identify what foods are "staples" in the book you're looking at pretty quickly and make up a shopping list.

7. When you are psychologically ready to tackle this, clean out everything you shouldn't eat from your pantry and fridge (unless others in your household are determined to continue eating those things). If you can't clean it all out, designate spaces in the pantry and the fridge so you can separate the healthy from the unhealthy. Don't even look at the unhealthy areas.

8. Fix some healthy things in large batches so they are ready and waiting for you the next time you're hungry. This will keep you from being unduly tempted by convenience foods that are unhealthy. Remember also that the healthiest way to prepare most fruits and veggies is raw. What could be easier?

9. There are new resources in development all the time at the Nutritional Health Education Center to help with this very issue, so check in regularly on the website (www.awesomehealthmakeover.com).

Controlling your environment

We have spent the whole chapter so far talking about what you eat and what you shouldn't eat. But there are other factors to consider under the heading of elimination.

One of the major categories of things you may need to eliminate consists of various media presentations which have never, until the last century, even existed in the human experience. It would be difficult to watch a sitcom based on the American experience 50 years ago and argue that the pace of life wasn't a lot slower back then. Go back 100 years and it's like another universe. The stress level in modern society has reached world record proportions and the result is that more people are now afflicted with some form of depression, anxiety, or personality disorder than ever before.

Step 2. News

We are bombarded daily with news from countries our ancestors didn't know existed. Worrying about what's happening in our own country is tough enough without worrying about a dozen others, too. The local evening news rarely has anything positive to report—it's always about the latest murders, thefts, and economic disasters. If you already have stressful events in your own life, such as health problems, listening to everybody else's troubles could push your stress-handling system over the edge.

A survey, compiled by Holmes and Rahe and first presented in the *Journal of Psychosomatic Research* in 1967, lists 43 ordinary events and gives them weight according to how stressful they are for your body. (www.actsweb.org/stress_test.php) Not all of these events would be considered negative by most people; they include such things as changing to a different line of work, buying a new house, having a new baby, or even retiring.

According to the survey, if you experience enough of these events in one year to earn a score of more than 300, you have an 80% chance of serious illness within the next 2 years. It takes only a few of these events to earn those 300 points. If our lives are so full of stresses that are real and largely unavoidable, we need to do all we can to minimize the stresses we can control.

The antidote to negative news is obvious. Stop watching it. Not only is it stressful, it typically comes at the worst possible time—right before bed when it may also cost you a good night's sleep. Lack of sleep amplifies the effects of stress tremendously. Chapter 4 is dedicated to a detailed discussion about sleep and why optimizing your sleep potential is a major key to unlocking your maximum health potential, but for now, just be aware that it is critically important.

On some level it's good to be informed, but you need to manage your news intake. Your coping ability is much greater in the morning, and morning news programs tend to report some informative and positive things along with the more troubling events. It may be wiser for you to go to bed earlier and get up early to enjoy some hot herbal tea and a little morning news instead. Maybe NPR on the way home from work or a quick look at the internet news headlines is what works for you. This is another area you must assess for yourself, but it is important to control and reduce media stress.

There are some things you cannot change, and knowing more about them doesn't really help you. We all need to focus on things that actually are within our sphere of influence. It's when we mentally resist what we can not change that we feel most stressed.

Addressing a problem you can actually solve usually decreases stress. By working on what we can change, we expand our sphere of influence and maybe eventually we can address those bigger issues. Your present smaller crises are the doors and windows through which you may someday reach out to impact the rest of the world. You have to use them to expand your circle one layer at a time—like rings in a tree. Like the tree, you have to grow into it.

Your next step is to consider how your news habits are affecting your life. If you could be doing better, plan how you will change this area of your life.

Step 3. Music

Many studies have been done on the effects of various frequencies on the body. The types of frequencies found in heavy metal music, for example, have been found to be stress producing while classical music frequencies are often soothing or mentally stimulating in a positive way. Other styles of music often fall somewhere in between.

Again, know thyself. Become aware of the effects of music on your body and mind. Listen to what supports you. You need not listen to classical music if you don't like it when there are so many other possibilities that have a positive impact. You owe it to yourself to explore them and find something you really do enjoy that also supports your health.

I will give you a personal example of the power of music over physiology from my own life. In my twenties I was going to a gym where they played loud rock music all the time. I usually listened to something a little softer or even some things much softer while not at the gym. I was in the habit of checking my heart rate after various exercises, and what I was seeing seemed higher than normal to me.

When I went jogging in my neighborhood, my heart rate stayed much lower than when I jogged the track at the gym. I paid attention to the level of tension in my body in both locations, and the only thing that stood out to me was the music. So I tried an experiment.

I took a Walkman with a tape of music I liked, which was not hard rock, and I listened to it while jogging at the gym. My heart rate was about 15 beats per minute slower. I tried it with and without my music and the results were consistent. The hard rock music elevated my heart rate by an average of 15 beats per minute every time. In terms of physiological stress, that's a huge difference! It can pay large dividends to control the media influence around you. For less than the price of poor seat at a single concert, an mp3 player allows you to control your listening anywhere, anytime.

Live music is also very powerful, and if you look around, you will probably find lots of local opportunities for live music—often for free. This is a very relaxing and enjoyable alternative to some less healthy forms of entertainment, such as violent movies…

Your next step is to consider how your music habits are affecting your life. If you could be doing better, plan how you will change this area of your life.

Step 4. Movies and video games

It seems like movie and game makers can't get enough violence these days. They are constantly finding ways to make it more realistic and graphic. What effect does this have on your nervous system? While some people are clearly more affected than others, everyone suffers ill effects on some level.

Many people believe that movie or video game violence doesn't matter because it's not real. While it's true that the human brain has a logic center to process that information, we also have less sophisticated areas of the brain designed for rapid, more emotional responses. These areas don't "think" logically. They do not know the difference. Some parts of your mind are affected by screen violence just as they would be if you saw it on the street and this is damaging to you in a number of ways.

If you habitually view graphic violence, you will, to some extent, become desensitized to human suffering and to the idea of causing it. For every action there is an equal and opposite reaction. With that loss of sensitivity, you will be less able to perceive and feel affection and compassion. This is damaging to good relationships with those who can offer you the emotional support you need to be healthy, and who need to receive that support from you. Do you even know what you're not giving or receiving?

I am not suggesting that you watch nothing but mushy, singing, purple dinosaurs, but I do think you need to be firmly in charge of your media experiences. We tend in this century to eat whatever passes in front of us and watch and listen to whatever goes on around us without thinking at all. I am suggesting that you eat, drink, watch, and listen purposefully and thoughtfully. Live on purpose, not by default. Manage your life; don't just let it happen to you.

Your next step is to consider how your visual media habits are affecting your life. If you could be doing better, plan how you will change this area of your life.

Step 5: Relationships

Even though it is necessary to eliminate things that hurt us, it is very hard to eliminate people who hurt us. Sometimes it is truly impossible. If you are dating an abusive person, you need to throw them out. Walk away and never go back. That's just all there is to it. If you have an abusive friend, you throw him out. Zero tolerance.

But what if you are married to someone who isn't supportive? What if it's a parent or a sibling? You can't throw them out without them taking a piece of your soul with them. My suggestion is to throw out the relationship, not the person.

Re-write the script you play out. Change you. Set some new boundaries—very strict ones. Protect yourself and your loved ones, and remember that taking good care of yourself is good for them, too. You can't be there for them if you are ill.

Relationships are a little like recipes. There are many ingredients, and if you change some of them, you have a completely different flavor—maybe a different dish altogether. You control 50% of the ingredients in every relationship you're a part of. When you change you, that's 50% of the recipe. It changes everything. You can't change another person, and the effort to do so damages relationships and causes stress for you. Change you.

People who really love you want you to take care of yourself—no exceptions. Sometimes they don't realize they are hurting or hindering you. It's okay to tell loved ones when and how they are hurting you, and it's okay to tell them what you need from them. Do it all in a loving, but firm way, and be prepared to stand your ground.

Sometimes people who love you don't understand what you are doing, and they really believe their abusive efforts to "save you" are for your own good. Educate them. Help them understand what you've chosen to do and why. Insist that they respect your right and responsibility to take care of your health.

Don't enable other people's bad habits by giving in to unhealthy pressure tactics, but don't constantly try to convert them to your way of thinking either—even if you really do know what's best for them.

Respect must go both ways or it really isn't respect at all. One-way respect is nothing but a power-trip. Don't fall for it. Your best defense against relationship stress is self-confidence. Give yourself the love you need, even if *they* don't. What do you wish they would do for you or say to you? Can you do that for yourself? Can you say it to yourself?

For more help on the subject of boundaries and relationships, I can think of no better resource than a book by Dr. Henry Cloud and Dr. John Townsend titled *Boundaries*.[6] If you have relationship stress, you should read the book and follow their advice.

A good relationship should be built on respect and trust—not on eating, wearing, or watching all the same things. If you reassure your difficult loved ones that your changes don't mean you love them any less or respect them any less, things should settle down.

Your next step is to consider how your relationships are affecting your life. If you could be doing better, plan how you will change this area of your life. Consider reading Boundaries.

Review

Key #3 Elimination

Eliminate What's Hurting You

Step 1: Take on the action plan for eliminating the 4 Fs from your diet.

Step 2: Review and adjust your news habits.

Step 3: Review and adjust your music habits.

Step 4: Review and adjust you visual media habits.

Step 5: Review and adjust your relationship boundaries.

Chapter 4: Sleep

We all know we need to sleep, but is it really that important to your health? Most Americans don't get an optimal amount of sleep and we seem to be getting along…but how many people do you know who are truly healthy? The average adult needs seven to eight hours of high quality sleep every night. How many people do you know who get that?

Studies show that when a person short-changes himself on sleep by as little as an hour or two each night, he is functioning like someone who is slightly drunk, and if you've ever experienced sleep deprivation, you know first-hand that it's true. Mental processing is slower, physical reaction time is slower, and there are other problems.

What does sleep have to do with any of that?

The night crew at work

We tend to think nothing happens while we're sleeping, but that isn't accurate at all. Just like in a big factory, different things happen on different shifts. To get a clearer picture of how sleep helps your body, think about your body as a factory.

In many factories, the night shift is an important time. With fewer people on the job using the equipment, it's an excellent opportunity for maintenance crews to inspect machines and make repairs. If there was never any down time, how could the equipment be kept in safe working order?

The janitorial staff, those unsung heroes, also do their best work at night while few people are about to get in the way. That's why everything looks in good order when you come in the morning ready to go to work.

Your body works the same way. During sleep, it is possible to grow and repair tissue at a faster rate than when you are awake due to resource allocation. Your body can't efficiently do everything all at once. Just as in the factory, you can't repair a machine that is still in full use; you need to at least slow it down.

The body also goes into a cleansing phase during sleep, detoxifying and taking out the trash while you aren't putting anything new in. If you don't get your sleep, your body won't have that "ready for action" look and feel in the morning.

But what about your mind? Compare the mind to a computer-based information-processing environment. During the day shift when computers and programs are in constant use with many workers inputting data, there is no convenient time to compile it all and organize it to be saved long-term. That will be done during off-hours when few people will be inconvenienced while the system is off-line.

The mind works the same way. You create memories all day long and make new mental connections. During the night, your short-term memory is processed to create long-term memory. That's one good reason not to cram for tests while staying up late the night before—you won't be able to remember much for long. Learning and remembering are much impaired by inadequate sleep. If you're wondering whether this is one way to help overcome memory problems, the answer is yes!

Additionally, the mind needs to process things emotionally so that you don't begin tomorrow with today's stress still hanging on. Dreams are one way emotions are processed—they are also one indicator of the quality of your sleep.

Lack of high quality sleep puts you at higher risk for every disease, all because of impaired functioning. It is well known that sleep deprivation increases risk for heart attacks, aggravates high blood pressure, worsens blood sugar control, makes it harder to control your weight, and even makes you a likelier candidate for cancer. Besides, it makes you cranky and you have no energy. I'm tired just thinking about it!

What is optimal sleep?

So, now that you're totally sold on the need to optimize your sleep, how would you define optimal sleep? There are three considerations: start time, quantity, and quality.

Start time is the easy one. Go to bed as close to 10:00 as possible. Hours of sleep that you get before 2:00 a.m. are twice as valuable as those you get later. It is much better to go to bed early and get up early than to stay up late when you need to get extra work done. We'll discuss how to determine precisely the best bedtime for you a little later.

The body goes through cycles which are based on many factors including sunlight, mealtimes, and habits. These factors work together to build a 24-hour cycle that helps your body function and get everything done. If you mess up the cycle, you suffer. Your body likes to eat, sleep, work, and play at the same times each day. Consistency is a great asset to your health.

• *Sunlight.* When the sun goes down, your body begins to wind down. This is accomplished hormonally. If you override that impulse to sleep, your hormones respond in such a way that may make it harder to get to sleep later. It is important to make these natural mechanisms work for you instead of fighting nature. Daylight Savings Time makes it hard for some people to stay well and sleep well through the winter. It helps to go to bed at least half an hour earlier in the winter to help your body accommodate the change.

• *Habits.* To revisit the factory analogy, your body has to "refit the machinery" for specific jobs through the day, and it learns to anticipate your habits. If you are accustomed to working out at a certain time each day, your body has learned to structure energy production around that and you may find it difficult to change. If you are accustomed to eating at 12:00 noon, changing to 1:00 p.m. may be uncomfortable for a while.

• *Mealtimes.* One of the cues your body uses to structure your biological cycles is the regularity of your mealtimes. If you've ever dealt with young children, you know that keeping mealtimes consistent goes a long way toward keeping nap times and bedtimes consistent and easy. It's still true when we're older; we just overcome it more gracefully. If an earlier bedtime is what you need, adjust your mealtimes to come a little earlier also, and be consistent.

Quantity

We've already established that most adults need seven to eight hours of quality sleep each night. That's pretty straightforward. There are a few who just can't stay asleep that long unless they're ill. If you're one of those, that's okay, but it is even more important for you to pay attention to quality and go to bed on time to make the most of the hours you can get.

Children need more sleep than adults. Increasingly, I see the disturbing trend of parents keeping children up late. Children's sports are running later than ever, and more and more parents are giving in to the pressure because "everybody's doing it."

Figure 1. How much sleep do you really need?

Age	Sleep Needs
Newborns (0–2 months)	12–18 hours
Infants (3–11 months)	14–15 hours
Toddlers (1–3 years)	12–14 hours
Preschoolers (3–5 years)	11–13 hours
School-age children (5–10 years)	10–11 hours
Teens (10–17 years)	8.5–9.25 hours
Adults	7–9 hours

I can't go out to a restaurant or a shopping center late at night without seeing exhausted, over-stimulated toddlers and even infants everywhere. This is very bad for a child's health. Immunity suffers with lack of sleep. A child's immune system is still developing and is challenged at every turn because the children are in schools, daycare centers, and play groups where they come into constant contact with a vast array of viruses and bacteria that are new to them. It just isn't fair to deprive a child of sleep.

The need for sleep changes as the child grows. Figure 1 is a fairly typical chart, prepared by the National Sleep Foundation (www.sleepfoundation.org), of suggested daily sleep times for people of all ages.

Now that you know about how much sleep you need, the question is when those hours should begin. Your perfect bedtime is unique to you, though probably very close to everyone else's. To determine the best time for you to go to sleep, observe your body's internal clock for a few days to see when, in the evening, you naturally feel a little wave of sleepiness.

When you do feel that "dip," you are feeling your natural sleep hormone, melatonin, kicking in. That's your body's way of telling you to fall asleep.

Be sure you choose a couple of quiet evenings for observational purposes. You may not feel the dip at all if you are over-stimulated.

If you usually feel that dip at 10:30, you should make a practice of being in bed with the light out by 10:20 so that when the feeling strikes, you can give in. In small children, the dip isn't always obvious, but the sign that you've passed it reads "hyper-activity." Little children accelerate when they're tired. Why?

When you feel the urge to sleep and you fight it off, what you're doing is recruiting your adrenal hormones to keep you awake. Adrenal hormones are stronger than melatonin, so they will keep you up, but the price you pay is adrenal fatigue and feeling lousy all the next day. Adrenaline rushes make kids appear hyper and causes poor impulse control, which is why they seem so cranky. The crankiness tends to catch up with adults the day after.

Sleep quality workshop

It is relatively easy to adjust your bedtime and the total amount of sleep you get, but sometimes quality is difficult to control. You don't have much influence once you fall asleep, but there are factors you can address before-hand that may have a significant impact on the quality of your sleep. These factors can be divided into two categories: your external environment and your internal environment.

External environment

We'll approach the issue of sleep quality in two parts. I'll walk you first through an overhaul of your external environment to help you eliminate things that might prevent a good night's rest. Get your pencil and clipboard and head for your bedroom. Really, get some paper, I'm serious. As we go through the following analysis of your sleeping space, make a list of changes you need to make, and then make them.

1. Purpose. Your bedroom needs to have purpose—a single purpose. It's for getting a good night's sleep in. If you work in here, or entertain yourself in here, or store all kinds of junk in here, you won't sleep well in here. You need to dedicate this space as a monument to peace and sleep, or at least make it look and feel that way.

   If you must work in the bedroom, try to arrange your workspace in an extra closet or behind a screen or curtain so that you can section it off from the sleeping zone. When its bedtime, you don't want to look at your workspace—it needs to look like a bedroom when you need one. Put work away at least an hour before you intend to sleep.

   Step 1, then, is to make sure you have a dedicated sleep space. Move your work to another room, and never ever work in bed. If that's impossible, make a curtain, buy a divider or an "office in a cabinet" and get busy on your redesign.

2. Excess clutter in the sleep zone is also a problem. An orderly, uncluttered space helps you relax. Clean up your room, and make sure that when you're done there is nothing left in here that doesn't help you feel safe, at home, and relaxed.

   Stacks of things that are awaiting your attention, work that needs doing, mail that needs sorting—all these remind you of stressful issues and possibly even feelings of guilt or failure. They should not be in your bedroom.

Sometimes even pictures of loved ones can be stressful. Personal belongings you have inherited may be painful reminders of someone you've lost, and you shouldn't have to deal with all of that when you are feeling tired and vulnerable. Be aware of how your belongings really affect you. Find a better place for things that cause emotional stress. Your bedroom is to be your personal oasis. It's where you go to get away from it ALL.. Take the time to make it your own.

Step 2 is to de-clutter your sleep space. Get a storage unit if necessary, have a yard sale, find a new place of honor for what is valuable but not helpful. Make your space sleek and uncluttered right away.

3. Décor. Consider all elements in your room—even the paint on the walls and the fabrics in the room. If everything looks too sterile or industrial, you may not achieve the soothing state of relaxation you want. If the colors are loud and stimulating, it may be time to redecorate. Reds, oranges, and yellows are very stimulating colors. For sleep enhancement, I would recommend softer, nearly neutral colors. Beige, soft blues or greens, or any light earth tones should be restful.

Step three is to make sure the design of your bedroom favors a good night's sleep. Re-paint or redecorate as necessary. A can of zero-voc paint is cheap; your health isn't. Go for it!

4. Mattress. Next, consider your mattress. If you are uncomfortable, you can't possibly sleep well. It may be time for something new. Although there are lots of newfangled options out there, they tend to be quite pricey and most fall short of the promises they advertise. For the most part, it's hard to beat a good old-fashioned mattress that's reasonably firm, yet soft to the touch. It's a worthy investment that can pay great dividends for years to come.

    If you are a very large person on a very small mattress, that's probably a mismatch worth correcting. If you aren't sleeping alone, make sure you have a mattress made for two. Sharing a very small mattress with somebody else can be a very big problem. If you are sleeping with a spouse who tosses and wallows, a bigger mattress may be essential for your comfort. Stressing the size of the bedroom is not nearly as bad as stressing your health, so opt for the bigger mattress if that helps you.

    Step four is to evaluate your mattress and optimize the size.

5. Bedfellows. Another consideration is that significant other over there. If he or she snores like a freight train in the moonlight, that must be

addressed. It is important to realize that snoring impairs the sleep of the guilty as much as the sleep of the innocent. Take your snoring spouse to an ear, nose and throat specialist to find out what is causing the snoring. It may be correctable, and that would benefit you both. Obviously, I don't favor cures that involve long-term use of steroids.

If the cause is not obvious or can't be corrected, try earplugs or any of several devices or methods of curing snoring and see if relief can be obtained. If he or she is willing, following all of the steps in the Awesome Health Makeover described in this book may bring relief through better health.

If your beloved snores or does other things that prevent you from sleeping deeply, and it can't be easily corrected, you may need to sleep separately, at least part of the time. I know, that's sacrilege to many, but even though sharing the night is a wonderful thing, if it means you leave him or her years before your time, it's not worth it.

An experiment may be necessary to determine how well you sleep *with*: try a night or two *without* and see how you feel. The guest room isn't such a bad place a few nights each week if you just really need to save your health.

A final word about those we sleep with. If you are co-sleeping with your child, you may need to consider transitioning the child to his or her own bed. Co-sleeping is a practice many mothers hold dear, and it is a decision you have to make for yourself. If your health is really on the line, however, you may not have the luxury of considering what is most agreeable to your maternal sensibilities. My advice is given with the feeling of one who has been there; don't sacrifice your days with your child for your nights. A toddler bed or crib can be placed right next to your own bed and that simple change can improve the quality of your sleep dramatically—if you can make peace with it.

In either case, remember the advice stewardesses give us on each flight: secure the oxygen mask to your own face BEFORE you attend to your child. If you're unconscious, or worse, you can't help the ones you love.

Step 5 is to honestly evaluate your co-sleeper and make adjustments.

6. Light. There are a couple more details in your physical environment that require your attention. One is the amount of light in the room while you are sleeping. Your hormonal system responds to light. Light wakes you; darkness encourages the release of hormones that help you sleep. Of course I'm speaking of melatonin.

Melatonin is the hormone that makes you feel sleepy at some point in the evening. If you manage it well, melatonin can be your ticket to a good night's sleep. Management is important and necessary, because we make less melatonin as we age. This is probably one of the reasons many elderly folk don't sleep as well, or as long, as they used to.

Melatonin isn't just good for sleep; it's a major hormone with an important role to play in overall hormonal balance, metabolism, and regulation of your entire circadian rhythm. There is evidence that it inhibits tumor growth and indirectly helps with many other conditions including fibromyalgia, depression, and migraine headaches.

Management of melatonin involves several steps, but for now, step one is to sleep in the dark—total darkness. Blocking as much light as possible from your sleeping quarters will help you maintain your melatonin level through the night and get a good night's sleep.

It is much better to keep a dim flashlight by your bed to illuminate your night-time adventures than to use a night-light. The same principle applies to your children. Night lights may ease fears while a child is falling asleep, but turn them off later. This should be an easy transition for all. Kids love flashlights, and you already know how to use one.

Even an excess of outdoor streetlights, car lights, or moonlight can interfere with your sleep. Room darkening drapes are the answer when outdoor light is the problem.

DVD players and digital clocks also produce light during the night. Repositioning, unplugging, or blocking the light from these appliances can also make a big difference if you are sensitive to light—and you don't know if you are until you try total darkness.

Step 6: Block light from your bedroom and get a cheap flashlight.

7. Electro-magnetic fields. Here's one almost no one thinks of—electro magnetic fields, EMFs for short. Because the body operates within its own EMF and uses EMFs for internal communication, your exposure to this energy can affect your health, and your sleep.

    It is best to remove electronic devices such as cell phones, clock radios, and such from the immediate vicinity of your bed. Keeping these devices out of the bedroom entirely is good, but at least move them far from your bed. You might even replace the plug-in model with a small battery operated clock—that doesn't tick.

    You also need to consider what is on the other side of the wall to which your head is nearest while sleeping. Is it an EMF-generating big screen TV or computer? You may need to move the appliance or the bed. Some of the most modern devices are remarkably good about not generating a huge field, but if in doubt, it won't hurt to move things around a bit.

Step 7: Manage your EMF exposure.

8. Temperature. Another factor to consider is your thermostat. In a house that is too warm or too cold, sleep may be disrupted by discomfort. Many people actually sleep better when the air is slightly cooler and the blankets warmer. It is worth a little experimentation to see what your optimal sleeping temperature is. It might save a bit on your electric bill as well!

   On a similar note, studies have shown that many people sleep better with pajamas and even socks than without. If you haven't experimented with this variable, it certainly is an easy thing to try.

   Step 8: Adjust your thermostat to see what temperature works best for you. If you're accustomed to sleeping au naturale, try some pjs and socks and see what happens. Do what works for you.

This completes the external environment workshop. Take your list and attack!

Internal environment

Now it's time for phase 2 of the sleep improvement workshop. Let's consider your internal environment. There are things going on within the body that affect sleep a lot. I can think of eight considerations that are within your control, some of which you've already addressed.

1. Caffeine. By now you should have successfully stopped the pop. If not, just do it. Coffee, tea, some granola bars, and other sources of caffeine need to be eliminated also if you are having sleep difficulties. All these caffeinated products are hard on your adrenal glands and so affect you on multiple levels.

   If you've already eliminated caffeine and unhealthy drinks, you may have already enjoyed a substantial improvement in your sleep. If you've eliminated them, but haven't replaced them with a good supply of water, that's your next step. Proper hydration helps your body relax and function. It also may help control some types of pain.

   Step 1 in managing your internal environment is to stop dehydrating and hyping up your body with caffeine and start hydrating properly. Refer back to chapter 2 for more help.

2.   Stress management. Addressing the root causes of your stress as mentioned in chapter one can make a big difference in your sleep. As discussed in chapter 3, some people simply can't work or think about stressful things close to bedtime and still get a good night's sleep. If you've already eliminated late-night stressful activities and you still have trouble sleeping, don't give up. There are still other things you can do to help.

If you've never considered meditation, you may want to give it a try. If you are a high stress person, you probably need help transitioning between your work life and your home life. Right after work, you probably find it difficult to change hats and become mom, dad, spouse, or whomever you need to be. Meditation, yoga, or tai chi might be just the ticket to a mental vacation from stress.

Far too many people leave work and go home only to shun the company of spouse and children for the solace of the TV or computer. Maybe this is how you attempt to transition. Is it working well for you? For your family? What if instead of two hours of TV, you could accomplish far more in twenty minutes of meditation? It's not a religion, it's just quiet contemplation, slower breathing, and getting in touch with yourself.

At work all day we listen to others and do for others and push our own needs and desires aside. It helps to set aside some time each day to listen to yourself—body and soul. It isn't about having specific thoughts or making any attempt to direct your thoughts. It's about taking time to breathe deeply and allow your mind to relax. This frees you to be who you want to be for the rest of your day.

There are lots of great books on meditation. Some are very complicated. They are nice, but I don't think they're necessary. If you just sit or lie down in a comfortable position, breathe deeply, allow your mind to unwind, consider what you are feeling and offer compassion to yourself, you will figure it out for yourself. Don't worry about doing it right—there is no wrong way as long as you aren't judging or controlling your thoughts.

For those who are more physical types, tai chi or yoga can be very much like a physical meditation. There are classes or videos from which you can learn the beneficial arts of tai chi or yoga. These are great stress relievers and all these methods carry the added benefits of helping you reduce your blood pressure and fatigue and keeping you mentally and physically balanced.

Step 2 is to be sure you have addressed your stress in a positive, proactive way.

3. Body mechanics. If you are the one who snores, you definitely need to address this issue. Go to the ENT doc, or a sleep clinic if necessary, to see what is causing the problem. Again, I don't like solutions that don't solve problems, so I'm not in favor of sleeping pills or steroids. It's always best to focus on the cause, not just on controlling or concealing symptoms. All the suggestions for a snoring spouse apply also to you.

   Weight issues can aggravate a snoring problem considerably. If you are significantly overweight, hang in there through the end of the book. There will be help for you to lose that weight, and your snoring and other sleep problems may disappear along with the unnecessary pounds.

   Step 3 is to address your own snoring issues if you haven't already.

4. Medication issues. Many medications affect the way people sleep. If you are taking medications for any reason, you should be aware that these may be altering your sleep patterns or otherwise affecting you.

   If you are having sleep problems, it would be a good idea to have a conversation with your medical doctor about the possibility that some of your medications may need to be adjusted or eliminated in order to improve your sleep. Don't fall prey, however, to the non-solution of adding a sleeping pill into the mix. That's not a good solution!

   A word of warning: please do not adjust or eliminate medications without the assistance of a medical doctor. If your doctor is uncooperative or dismissive, get a new one. Ask around for recommendations about doctors in your area who respect your wishes and listen to you. They are out there; sometimes they're just a little hard to find.

   Step 4 is to enlist your doctor to help you adjust medications which may be interfering with your sleep.

5. Pain management. Pain is keeping a lot of people up at night these days. If you are one of them, a visit to your local chiropractor might bring blessed relief. You might be surprised how many conditions fall within the scope of chiropractic care.

   Because chiropractic procedures focus on the spine and the musculoskeletal system, they focus, by extension, on the nervous system. There is no bodily function that occurs outside the influence of the nervous system, so there really is no physical condition which cannot be more efficiently addressed when you are correctly adjusted by a chiropractor.

Chiropractic adjustment restores function and balance to your nervous system. What condition could you have in which you would not benefit from your nervous system functioning as well as it can?

Some people are afraid of chiropractors. They fear bones will be broken, maybe even in their neck. In the statistical realm of medical mistakes, the number of people who have suffered serious injury due to chiropractic mistakes or accidents is extremely low. The probability of such a mishap during surgery or drug administration is statistically much higher.

Additionally, many chiropractors are trained to use a small device called an activator. For the truly timid, this is an excellent alternative to the "neck wrenching" style of manipulation that some people fear. The activator is placed along your neck and you hear a little click and feel a very light little thump, like someone flicking you. It is completely safe. Many chiropractors use these, especially if you ask them to.

You shouldn't allow fear of chiropractic to keep you from doing what you need to do for your health. The odds of your being injured in a car accident on the way to the chiropractor's office are at least a thousand times greater than your odds of being injured in his office. You don't shy away from the dentist or MD for fear of mistakes; why should you do so with your chiropractor who, statistically, makes far fewer of them?

Step 5 is to find a good chiropractor and get an adjustment. You need your nervous system working for you, not against you.

6. Hormonal regulation. If you fall asleep easily but wake often in the night, you may have blood sugar regulation issues. If your blood sugar falls too low during the night, adrenal hormones will come to your rescue. A surge of adrenal hormones is like taking an espresso IV. It will wake you up and keep you up a while. It is worthwhile to have your blood sugar checked if staying asleep is a big problem.

In the meantime, try having a small, light late-night snack to help get you through the night. A handful of fresh nuts or seeds such as almonds, sunflower seeds, or pumpkin seeds is a healthy snack—just please avoid the oily or salty ones. Keeping these by your bed in case you need a little something during the night may also be helpful.

The flip-side to this is that having too much food to process during the night can mean feeling tired the next day. When you eat too much late night food, your mind sleeps, but your body doesn't—it has to work half the night digesting your midnight snack. If you need a late-night snack to get through the night, keep it light. Raw food digests much more easily and quickly than cooked food, so it's a better choice late at night.

Step 6 is to make sure your blood sugar is under control and take steps to correct it if it isn't.

7.   Supplements. I am reluctant to mention this here for fear you will skip to this step prematurely. As a last resort, it may be necessary to use a supplement or two to achieve deep, restful sleep. If you are desperate, or under much pressure from a family member or doctor, however, you need this information now.

I encourage you strongly to make every effort to achieve good sleep by means of healthful living before resorting to supplements which may be difficult for you, emotionally or hormonally, to wean off of later. Mastering all of the other 6 keys is the best way to get your sleep under control. But if you must...

Try some supplemental melatonin. This is the hormone your body produces naturally to help you sleep. If your production is low, you may need this help. All the other suggestions in this book might, in time, help restore your natural production nearer to normal and that is why I encourage you to do everything else first.

If you are going to try melatonin, do it right. Use a liquid preparation for better absorption. Start with the lowest possible dose, don't use more than you need, and use it consistently.

Taking melatonin successfully is largely a matter of timing. If you didn't already do so, observe your body's internal clock for a couple of days to see when, in the evening, you naturally feel a little wave of sleepiness. As we discussed before, when you feel that little "dip," what you are feeling is your natural melatonin kicking in—your body's way of telling you to go to sleep.

If you feel that dip at 10:30, you should be in bed with the light out by 10:20 so that when the feeling strikes, you can blissfully surrender. If you are not going to obey your internal commands, supplemental melatonin probably won't help you anyway.

Once you've determined your correct bedtime, based on your natural release of melatonin, take your supplemental melatonin to coincide with your natural release—about 15 minutes before you try to fall asleep. Once you've taken it, don't fight it. Go to bed immediately.

When you feel the urge to sleep and you fight it off, remember that you're recruiting your adrenal hormones to keep you awake. Adrenal hormones are stronger than melatonin, so they will keep you up, but the price you pay is adrenal fatigue and feeling lousy the next day.

If you are going to try melatonin, please be aware that it is not meant for occasional, symptomatic use. It is a hormone and it needs to be used consistently to get good results. Use it for a month to see if it will help before you decide it doesn't work for you.

If you want something for occasional stress-related insomnia, melatonin isn't a good choice. Try some chamomile or valerian as an extract or a tea for the occasional difficult evening.

Step 7 is to be used as a last resort. Try supplements if absolutely necessary. For persistent insomnia, try melatonin first, since it is naturally occurring and conveys other health benefits. For occasional trouble try chamomile or valerian.

8. Finish this program. If you implement all the suggestions in this and the preceding chapters and still have trouble sleeping, don't despair. There are still three more chapters, and the work you do in those chapters will also help you achieve sound sleep. The 7 Keys are inter-related.

    It takes faith to continue when progress is slow, but don't give up. Success comes to those who persevere. You will learn about the effects of proper breathing, diet, and exercise in the upcoming chapters, and all of these elements will affect your sleep significantly.

    Although there are obviously lots of ways to address sleep directly, to some extent, good sleep will remain a work in progress until your program is complete.

    Step 8: Finish the book and implement all of the AWESOME Health Makeover.

Bedtime routine

The final section of this chapter is good for everyone, regardless of how well you sleep now. Establishing a bedtime routine can help someone who sleeps poorly sleep better, but it can also improve sleep for those whose sleep is already high quality, and it helps prevent problems from developing.

A bedtime routine helps you unwind and tells your body what to prepare for. It is extremely helpful for those who do sleep well, but may have a little trouble falling asleep initially. You should not have to linger awake in bed more than 15 minutes from the time you get into it before you fall asleep—ideally.

The components of your routine will be unique, but what matters is that you are consistent. Common elements include taking your dog out for his final evening constitutional, turning out lights in the main part of the house, checking door locks, putting on pjs, brushing and flossing teeth, etc.

These are fine things to do before bed, but if you are having trouble sleeping or going to sleep, there are a few things you might need to stop doing.

• Dimming lights in the house half an hour before bed can make a difference in stimulating natural melatonin production and helping you wind down. Turning off the computer and TV at least an hour before bed can help also. Restricting the activities of your last waking hour of each evening to very quiet pursuits can be extremely helpful.

• Do some tai-chi. Read an enjoyable book—not a professional journal that makes you think about work. Talk quietly with family members—about things you agree on. Write cards to friends. Take a relaxing bath with lavender bath salts. Listen to relaxing music. The possibilities are sweet. Enjoy them.

• If you feel stressed by what lies ahead tomorrow, check your schedule, make up your to-do list, and put your desk in order—before your quiet hour. This will allow you to take your brain offline without fear that you will forget something important.

• If you do everything "right" and yet find yourself unable to fall asleep, or if you wake in the night and are unable to return to sleep, don't fight that either. It is better to get up for a little while and try again a little later than to lie miserably in bed because you will associate that misery to your sleep space and it could become habitual. Just do something quiet in dim light for a little while, and avoid stimulating activities.

It's a good idea to actually write down your basic night-time ritual. There is a lot to remember. To some extent it may consist of a list of options you want to explore, but knowing what you will do is half the battle. Allowing time for what you have to do before bed is the key to getting there on time. Be kind to yourself and be consistent.

Final step: install a healthy bedtime routine to optimize your sleep potential.

Review

Key #4 Sleep

Optimize your sleep potential

Step 1: Figure out how much sleep you need.

Step 2: Find your ideal bedtime.

Step 3: Adjust your external environment.

Step 4: Adjust your internal environment.

Step 5: Install your bedtime routine.

Chapter 5: Oxygen

You can get by without food for weeks, water for days, but you can't live five minutes without oxygen. Why is that? Your body is running more chemistry experiments every hour than the three biggest chemical manufacturers in the country, combined. Everything you do, and even your continued existence in living form, depends completely on all those chemical reactions taking place in your body. You can't even blink your eyes without chemistry. Oxygen is required—no substitution is possible—for nearly *all* of those reactions.

Your body, your laboratory, your factory...

You are a veritable factory. Every day you have to make stomach acid, saliva, proteins, sweat, hormones, enzymes, energy, new body cells, and many other products to keep your internal world humming. You need ingredients for all that chemistry, and oxygen is without question one of the most heavily used ingredients in your internal laboratory. Without it, things just shut down.

What kind of things shut down? You know that if oxygen is not delivered to your brain, you'll pass out in just a minute or two. Your cells are the same way. They begin to suffer immediately in the absence of oxygen. It's not realistic to list things that shut down—everything does. This is as true in the body as in a factory during a power failure. What systems lose power? All of them! The computers in the office, the big machines on the floor, the conveyor belts, even the janitor's vacuum cleaner—they all stop because they can't move without power.

In chemistry, oxygen is power. So many of our necessary chemical reactions are oxidation-driven that we can't live without it for more than a couple of minutes.

We use oxygen to burn food for fuel. Did you ever blow on a fire to make it burn hotter? Have you ever seen what happens to the fire when no air gets to it? How long does it take to put out a fire in the absence of oxygen? It's instantaneous. It just stops burning.

We use oxygen in oxidation reactions to destroy invading organisms like bacteria and viruses. Oxidation reactions are also used to disarm toxins in the bloodstream, as they pass through your liver.

The two primary causes of all disease are toxicity and deficiency. Both of these are utterly inescapable without an ample supply of oxygen. It's like being under siege and getting bombed at the same time. You're done.

Since oxygen is so important, how we get it really matters, and there are multiple sources. If you look at the chemical formulas for food and water, you see that oxygen is present in all of them. Of all the food you could eat, fresh fruits and vegetables have the most abundant supply of oxygen. The amount of oxygen available from all foods decreases as we cook them, so there is another good reason to eat more raw food.

The mechanics of breathing

Clearly however, the primary source of oxygen is the air we breathe. While we can't control the chemistry occurring in our lungs, we can control the mechanical process that brings the air in there. Breathing seems like a simple thing and we all do it already, but there are distinct advantages for those who learn to do it better.

Because it is one of your automatic functions and you don't have to think about it, most people don't really know how breathing actually works. Understanding the basic physiology of breathing is very helpful. The key players are your two lungs and your diaphragm.

Your lungs are like two balloons and your diaphragm is a sheet of muscle that lies right underneath them. Your diaphragm separates your body cavity into two halves. Your respiratory and circulatory organs are in the top half and your digestive organs are in the bottom half.

When you breathe properly, you pull your diaphragm down lower in your gut, your lungs expand to fill the extra space in your chest, and they take in air. As your diaphragm goes down and your lungs begin to expand, your lower rib cage expands from front to back and from side to side, bringing fresh air into the deepest regions of both lungs. Finally, the diaphragm relaxes to its original position and releases the air back out.

In between the drawing of air in and the releasing of air back out, a lot of chemistry happens in the lungs and the bloodstream. All of your blood follows a closed circuit of blood vessels all over the body that is completed every minute or two. As it passes through the intricate network of tiny vessels in your lungs, gasses are exchanged. Carbon dioxide diffuses out of your blood vessels and into the air spaces in your lungs to be expelled, while oxygen from the lungs diffuses into the bloodstream to be carried to the rest of the body.

Breathing happens. Whether you are doing it on purpose or not, your nervous system constantly monitors the process. If you get distracted and stop thinking about your breathing, your nervous system will switch your breathing controls seamlessly to autopilot. That switch can be a blessing or a curse, depending on your habits.

Your breathing habits

What sort of habits do you have? Millions of people have forgotten what a proper deep breath feels like. In our high-stress world, many people are so tense they never take a deep relaxed breath. You can draw air in two different ways—expanding your upper rib cage, or drawing your diaphragm down as described earlier.

For many people, the diaphragm moves very little. The lower ribs remain stationary, and the upper chest expands to fill only the top part of the lungs. The air in the bottom portion of the lungs remains stagnant and oxygen-depleted, which means that the lowest third of your lung area is essentially not used, and thus not "cleaned out."

One of the underappreciated aspects of vigorous breathing is that it helps to remove old mucus from the lungs. It is possible to have considerable accumulation of debris in the lower lungs for years which creates an environment ripe for infections such as pneumonia to take hold.

We all know how it feels to have a sudden temporary reduction of air intake, but many people have lived years with a chronic shortage and don't really know what they're missing. Like poor eyesight, poor breathing can creep up on you.

How important is technique in breathing? Technique influences how much oxygen you take in and thus, how well saturated your tissues are with oxygen.

Some facts about oxygen and cancer

Oxygen saturation is important for everyone, but if your family has a history of cancer, it may be especially important for you. More than 50 years ago, Professor Otto Warburg of the Kaiser Wilhelm Institute for Biology—a German physiologist, medical doctor, and Nobel laureate—discovered that while your healthy body cells are dependent on oxygen, cancer cells don't use it so much. They are partially or completely anaerobic. In fact, cancer cells can not thrive in a well-oxygenated environment. Is this the ultimate cure for cancer? No, but I do want to be sure that every cubic inch of my body is well oxygenated if it helps me fight cancer any better.

A little-known fact about cancer is that in a very real sense everyone already has it. Abnormal cells are produced every day by every body. They are nothing more or less than your own normal cells which have been damaged. There are an infinite number of ways to damage a cell, but the immediate result is that the damaged cell's inability to manage oxygen properly is a core problem.

Remember that every cell is dependent on oxygen the same way a modern factory depends on electricity. If the life of the cell is to continue, a back-up power source has to be found fast. When oxygen is in short supply, cells can begin meeting some of their power needs through fermentation—making acids. They can run on that—but just enough to survive and reproduce, not enough to do ANY of their other regular jobs. It's a scary sacrifice for a cell to make, but they do it as a leap of faith, hoping conditions will improve so they can go back to being normal productive members of your internal society.

According to Warburg's research, for the first few days, the damage may be reversible; but if the cell doesn't restore normal respiration soon, the change becomes permanent. If oxygen supply is restored within those first hours or days, the cell may normalize and heal. If not, either the cell will die, or it will live on as a cancer cell. Survivor cancer cells are not usually a problem because a healthy immune system will destroy them. But when your immune system has been weakened and you have created a favorable environment, these cancer cells may form a whole colony. That's when they become a problem.

Yeasts, bacteria, and you

It's a similar situation with bacteria and yeasts. We all have them, all the time, and some are even beneficial. But one thing really stands out: generally speaking, the bad guys hate oxygen and love sugar. Health is about keeping everything in balance; it's a numbers game.

We need to keep the home court advantage by making sure our home court supports us—not the enemy. We can't allow our internal conditions to favor the growth of cancers, bacteria, and yeasts. We have to control our own biological terrain. In the war for health, these 7 Keys will help you take your body back and keep control of it for the rest of your life.

Terrain is everything....they don't come until they're called.

The fact that these offenders are always around is the reason we have to concern ourselves with maximizing our health all the time, not just occasionally. Bacteria, viruses, and cancer cells are actively working against you every minute, and they are extremely opportunistic. If you provide them any opportunity, they'll take it. They never miss a trick.

A well-known forerunner of modern medicine, Claude Bernard, is credited with having made the provocative statement: "The terrain is everything; the germ is nothing." This means that you are only as vulnerable to disease as you allow yourself to be. Your susceptibility to any germ, fungus, bacteria, or cancer cell is dependent on whether your internal environment will support the life of the invading organism.

Another famous saying often repeated in alternative medicine circles is that "flies don't cause garbage." I personally like to say "fleas don't attract dogs." Either way, the point is that pathogenic invaders are attracted to what feeds them. If you leave trash on your back porch, you must expect to be visited by possums, raccoons, and rodents. If you leave trash in your body, you must expect to be visited by bacteria, viruses, and yeasts. They don't come until they're called. You call them by how you maintain, or fail to maintain, a strong healthy internal environment, and if you keep feeding them, they stay and reproduce.

Oxygen, breathing, and stress management

Stress management is another major issue related to breathing and oxygen intake. Have you ever narrowly avoided a bad car accident? How did your breathing change? When you have a sudden shock you breathe in a gasping fashion high in your chest. Your diaphragm isn't much involved. This response is so universal you can recognize it visually if you see someone react this way. You know it means they are shocked or afraid. They are on alert.

Communication experts tell us that 70% of all communication is non-verbal—ironically, we call it "body language." I say ironically, because "body language" is exactly what we use to communicate with our own bodies. Your body speaks body language fluently. When you breathe high in your chest without using your diaphragm, your body says, "Uh-oh, we're in danger!"

The adrenal glands respond immediately, because they exist to help us in times of crisis by cranking out fight-or-flight hormones. When you really are in danger, these hormones are essential to your survival. When you aren't, they're a major hindrance to your well-being.

Fight-or-flight hormones cause changes in your body chemistry that affect blood sugar control, blood pressure, heart function, and pretty much every system in your body. When they are in circulation in quantity, these hormones put your body in a "stress-response" state. That's okay for a few minutes, but it's terrible when it becomes a lifestyle!

Can something as simple as breathing cause your blood pressure to stay up, your depression or panic attacks to worsen for long periods of time, your digestion to be poor, your heart rate or rhythm to malfunction, your hormones to be out of balance, your weight to increase…? Yes, it can!

Fortunately, we can also purposefully use body language to tell our bodies all is well, "stand down red alert." We have to breathe correctly. When you breathe correctly you tell your body it's okay.

One final aspect of breathing mechanics you need to know about is how your breathing affects your lymphatic system. Most people know little about the lymphatic system, yet it is vital to your health.

It consists primarily of fluid, which is mostly water, surrounding your cells. It's like the neighborhood your house is in. The street out front is the nearest blood vessel and delivery trucks represent all that the blood stream and the blood cells deliver to the door of each cell every day as well as the garbage trucks that carry away the trash. The space the garbage man or the delivery man has to pass through to get to your door is the lymphatic fluid.

A delivery man or garbage man can walk right up to your door, but nutrients and wastes don't have legs or a mind of their own. How do they get from the street to the door?

Have you ever put a drop of food coloring into a bowl of water? As long as the water is still, the drop of color sits there and doesn't spread very much. If you stir the water, the color spreads fast to fill all the water in the bowl. This is how your lymphatic system works. When you move your muscles, the fluid moves and the nutrients and wastes get transported. If you don't move, lymph fluid doesn't either. Cells don't get nutrients, including oxygen, and don't get their wastes carried away either, at least not efficiently.

Your blood has a pump—your heart—to move your blood around your body. Your lymph fluid has no pump. It moves as you move—and as you breathe. The nearest thing to a pump for your lymphatic system is your diaphragm. When you take a nice deep breath using your diaphragm, your rib cage, your back, and abdominal muscles, most of the lymph fluid in your body cavity around all your major organs gets moved.

This is one reason exercise is healthful and stress reducing. It makes you breathe deeply. It's even one reason, apart from the intense addiction, smokers feel like they "need" a cigarette. When they get tense, their breathing becomes very shallow and their adrenals are on alert. When they light up, what's the next thing they do? Yep, a nice slow, deep breath. "Ahhh, cough, cough…"

Whether you are wheelchair bound, bed-ridden, or just chained to your desk you can probably do breathing exercises to enjoy many of the health benefits of exercise.

Breathing correctly

Now that you're convinced you need to learn how to breathe correctly, let's assess your breathing to see where you are right now. It's really simple.

Lie on your back and place one hand on your chest and the other hand on your belly button. Breathe normally. Which hand is going up and down the most? If the hand on your chest is moving the most, you've just diagnosed yourself as a chest breather. If the hand on your stomach moved more, you are primarily an abdominal breather. Well done.

If you are a chest breather, you can re-learn how to breathe, and it will make a big difference in how you handle stress and how your body functions for you.

If you already breathe correctly, you can strengthen and improve your capacity and control to improve your health further and manage stress more purposefully.

In either case the following exercise is what I recommend for everyone. It is good maintenance and preventive care for your body and mind. If you are not already breathing correctly, you should practice this exercise as many times daily as you can to keep your breathing in your conscious mind. As you do so, it will become more habitual. Be patient, because this could take weeks, especially if you have asthma. It may be helpful to practice with your hand (or a favorite toy for a child) on your stomach so you can monitor whether you are doing it correctly.

A correctly drawn breath has four parts which should flow smoothly and seamlessly in the following order:

1. Inhale to fill the belly
2. Inhale to expand the lower ribs
3. Exhale to release from the rib cage
4. Exhale to release from the belly

Basic Breathing Exercise

1. Lie down, or sit up straight without crossing your legs. Close your eyes, relax your mind, and drop your shoulders. Take a <u>slow</u> deep breath in to the count of 5 (one one-thousand, two one-thousand). Be sure to inflate the belly first, then the lower rib cage.

2. Hold the breath to the count of 5 as above.

3. Release the breath to the count of 10 in reverse order—rib cage first, then the belly.

4. Repeat this process 10 times (10 breath cycles).

Don't be tempted to be impatient; each cycle of breath takes only 20 seconds. Even 200 seconds for the whole exercise is less than 3 ½ minutes. You deserve at least that much time dedicated to your health.

Remember some of the benefits deep breathing while you breathe:

*   Lowers blood pressure
*   Reduces tension and anxiety
*   Assists in weight loss
*   Helps prevent cancer and infection
*   Aids in recovery from cardiovascular disease
*   Helps improve digestion and metabolism
*   Increases energy level
*   Helps cleanse the body
*   Helps you think more clearly

Completing this exercise at least 3 times each day should lead to measurable increases in blood oxygen even after only a few days of practice. As you do it more, correct breathing habits will become a way of life even when you are not actively doing a breathing exercise.

Try making it a habit immediately before meals to improve digestion, and at bedtime to promote a restful night's sleep. Your nervous system has two "gears," one for things like eating and sleeping, one for thinking and working. If you are in "working gear" you won't be set up to digest food or sleep well. If you are in "eat/sleep gear" it will be hard to get much done.

Using the breathing exercise helps you downshift from working mode to eating or sleeping mode which helps your digestion and sleep efforts. Don't try to reverse this and chest breathe to wake yourself up, however, as it just makes you anxious and aggravates all those problems listed above.

The art of breathing properly is not widely recognized, but the lack of it in our culture is obvious. Improper breathing aggravates so many diseases and correcting this key to health is so easy. Everyone should master this one.

Review

Key #5 Oxygen

Optimize your breathing and your oxygen potential.

Step 1: Assess your current breathing technique.

Step 2: Begin doing the breathing exercise at least 3 times daily.

Chapter 6: Maximize Your Nutrition

Part 1. What Is Eating Really About, Anyway?

Is diet a stressful topic for you? Are you sick and tired, literally, from trying to figure out what to eat every time you get hungry; never feeling sure you're doing the right thing? Always worrying you might be doing more harm than good? Just tired of having to think about it when no one else does? Ugh!

Take a deep breath and let all that stress go. It's over. This chapter is just for you. In chapter 3 we discussed things you need to eliminate, and hopefully you've been working on that. With all of those eliminations behind us, we can now afford to address maximum nutrition from a more positive point of view. The idea is to make eating simple and stress-free once again.

Removing the stress from our diet

Stress is a symptom of something called cognitive dissonance. Cognitive dissonance is a fancy term meaning lack of harmony in the mind. Stressed is how you feel when you have beliefs that conflict with each other, or when your actions are not in alignment with your beliefs.

When you want to change something but you don't follow through, it's generally because you have a conflict between the new actions you're trying to take and the old beliefs you're still hanging on to. You want the change, but you're not buying the new story you're telling about why you need it. You are wanting something else that comes with an easier, more familiar story. Sometimes we also feel like it's just not fair. "Why should I have to watch what I eat? Nobody else does and they're doing all right..." New actions need new beliefs to drive them, but they can be so hard to install.

If you are like most people, you believe that eating right is necessary for good health on some level, but you also believe that it isn't always necessary or that there are alternatives to it such as exercise. You probably also have a constant inner debate running about what constitutes eating right—you're probably most eloquent and persuasive when you want something that isn't very good for you.

When you were a kid, eating probably wasn't stressful. You probably didn't think about it much at all. The stress came later as you learned more about health. But there were lots of beliefs that took root in those early carefree years, and they are what's giving you such a hard time now. Your newer beliefs may be more accurate, but the old ones are stronger because they've been there longer.

Your food identification system

The core issue is your food identification system. If you can change what you identify as food, your temptation level, and your stress, will be much lower. Remember that we take actions based on our strongest beliefs. If your beliefs are right, your actions will be right most of the time also. With that in mind, let's assess the belief system you already have.

Why don't you reach for a trash can or a flower pot when you're hungry? You probably did when you were very young, but somebody told you that was yucky and it would make you sick. You don't currently identify those things as food, because you believe they will make you sick. You don't have to think about it constantly, you just know. Avoiding trash cans and flower pots when you're on the prowl for food is effortless for you now because early in life you linked the fridge and the pantry with the idea of feeling full and healthy, and you linked those other things with the image of sickness.

Later on, you learned that when you were hungry there were sources of food all around you. Vending machines, fast food restaurants, the ice cream truck, coworkers bearing donuts… it's everywhere—if you identify that stuff as food. The point is, there was a time in your life when you didn't see it as food and you didn't look for it.

Changing beliefs to create the change you need

It was a major shift in my thinking, but now when I'm hungry, I literally don't see fast food stores or vending machines as food options any more than the nearest bank or post office. There is no food there! How do you make a shift like that happen? It's a matter of changing your beliefs.

Beliefs are based on acquired knowledge and repetitive reinforcement. Once you understand what your body needs and where it comes from, you can change your definition of food. With practice, you can learn new habits. Greater knowledge and practice are what it takes to go from driving past a fast food store feeling sorry for yourself to driving past feeling proud of yourself to not even noticing it at all. The following are three core beliefs that are required to drive this kind of change:

1. You really have to believe that what you eat matters. Until I truly believed junk food would hurt me, I couldn't give it up. For an exercise in continuous reinforcement, from now on when you go to the grocery store, play the cart game. It isn't really a game, it's actually a serious exercise in which you discreetly scope out other people's carts to see what they're buying.

Consider the person pushing the cart. What can you learn about the results this diet produces? It won't take you long to spot somebody who looks miserably unhealthy pushing a basket full of frozen dinners, chips, pop, and donuts. Maybe they're on a riding cart, maybe they're carrying an oxygen tank. When you see this person, you'll probably feel a wave of compassion, maybe even sadness. But he or she has something important to teach you. You give at least a little meaning to their suffering when you learn from them and say to yourself, "Yes, I believe that what I eat really does matter."

2. You have to believe *this* meal matters, and tell the truth. Frequently, we accept our inferior actions by rationalizing that it's "just this once." We all know it's *not* just once; it's really a habit. Habits are changed one action at a time. Each time you bite the bullet instead of the burger and take the time to do it right, you learn ways to do it better, easier, and faster next time. Take the time to find better food choices—every time you get hungry.

3. You have to believe you're worth the extra effort of finding real food. Honestly, we put ourselves down just for convenience. If your child were not well, would you make him or her eat something junky just because you were a little short on time? Love would not allow you to do that. You have to love yourself that way. If it helps, remember you're also doing it for them—they need you to be well for them for a long time yet.

You have to re-educate yourself and install a new mindset, then you can step back and let it work for you. When you were very young, you learned dozens of facts about health and nutrition that kept you alive up to this point, but they probably weren't accurate or thorough enough to keep you thriving well into your 90s, or to help you make good decisions when there is so much conflicting information bombarding you on a daily basis.

Knowledge is power—the power to make right decisions. Knowledge about how your body works and what it needs is essential to a solid decision-making process. The following is a crash course to give you some powerful reasons to create some new beliefs about food—and make them stick.

Nutrition 101

Jumping in at the deep end of the pool, how is it possible that we could even have disease in a self-healing body? And why am I asking that question in a section on nutrition? Let's define these terms: degenerative disease, anabolism, and catabolism.

- Anabolism—building new tissue by making new cells.
- Catabolism—breaking down old tissue; older cells are dying.
- Degenerative disease—old cells are dying faster than you can replace them with new ones.

If you didn't really process those terms, please, go back for a second look.

These words represent very important concepts in health, and their relationship to nutrition is profoundly significant. When your old cells are dying faster than new ones are being born, we say you are in a catabolic state. If the opposite is true and you are building up, healing, getting better, you are in an anabolic state.

Athletes are often tempted to take anabolic steroids. These make you grow more muscle and other tissue, and they speed up the healing process. That's where the unfair advantage issue comes from, and that's why it's often illegal.

When you stay in a catabolic state for a long time, the result is degenerative disease. Cancer, diabetes, heart disease—all of the major scourges of our time—are degenerative diseases.

You don't need steroids to be in a mildly anabolic state that favors healing, but what do you need? If your car breaks down, you can't fix it unless you get some new parts to replace the broken ones. When your body breaks down, you have to grow new cells to replace the old broken ones. What are new cells made of and where can you get some?

Macro versus micro nutrients

The old saying, "you are what you eat" wasn't far from the truth. Unlike plants, which are capable of producing their own food "in house," humans have to eat. There are two classes of nutrients, macro and micro.

Macro nutrients are the big, broad categories: protein, fat, and carbohydrate. Micro nutrients are cofactors in nutrition, namely vitamins, minerals, and phytonutrients. For the most part, macro nutrients are either burned as fuel or used as building material. If you burn it, that's measured in calories. A calorie is like an inch or a quart. It's just a measurement to describe the burn-ability of a food, not an ingredient in the food.

Enzymes—the workers in your body

When new tissue (new cells) is built in your body, what does the work of building? Building occurs from within your cells. One cell duplicates all of its inside parts, splits into two cells, and then starts over again.

To make that happen, millions of chemical reactions must occur. Those reactions are facilitated by enzymes. Enzymes are like little robotic workers. Each one has a job to do—generally either putting two things together or taking two things apart. Each enzyme work-bot also has a battery pack that turns him on or off. That battery pack is a micro nutrient—a vitamin or a mineral.

If a micro nutrient battery pack (cofactor) is missing, an enzyme gets turned off and does not do its job *at all*. Each enzyme is capable of performing its function 40,000 times—*per second!* There are millions of enzymes in your body requiring those nutrients every second. That's a lot of vitamins and minerals you need and a lot of down time when you don't get enough. You can definitely see how this is relevant to the nutrition discussion.

When you wake up every morning and head off to work, your cells are hard at work too. Their work is to make the energy you use to do your work. Do you get tired around 3:00 or 4:00 every afternoon? If you run out of steam, your cells aren't keeping up with your energy demands. How do cells make energy? Oddly enough, it's called cellular respiration. It's the burning of sugar to produce energy. It's called respiration because oxygen is involved to help light the fire.

Energy production—a very simplified view

In the mitochondria of each cell, one molecule of sugar at a time enters an energy producing cycle of chemical transformations. Think of it like a circular assembly line with more of those enzyme work-bots at each station. In the beginning of the cycle, a carrier molecule escorts an already altered sugar molecule into the cycle. At each station, the molecule complex is altered by a different enzyme and a tiny bit of energy (called ATP) is released in the process. The molecule moves on to the next station and another change is made and a little more energy is released. This process continues until the carrier molecule that started the cycle is restored to its original form so that it can pick up another sugar and go around again, ideally.

There is a fly in the ointment. What happens if one of the micronutrient battery packs is missing and one enzyme work station is shut down? The process stops right there. Instead of 38 units of energy being produced in this cycle, maybe we only get up to 15 units. The carrier is not ready to re-enter the cycle. We also have a lot of partially processed bits and pieces floating around. It's not a clean or efficient process, is it? Kind of like driving a car that gets really bad gas mileage and smokes a lot.

That's what it's like when you don't have all the vitamins and minerals you need. That's why we can easily fall into a state of disrepair—catabolic degenerative disease. Like a construction crew sleeping on the job, you can't build much without sufficient energy and materials.

H=7k The total health equation

In an excellent book called *Eat to Live*,[2] Dr. Joel Fuhrman explains that Health = Nutrients / Calories. This is his "equation of health," and it's a great way to summarize some key points in nutrition.

While I would not hesitate to recommend *Eat to Live*, I would love to tweak his equation. I believe that Maximum Nutrition = Nutrients / Calories. I believe health depends not only on nutrition, but on all 7 Keys. My own equation would look like this: H = 7K. That stands for "Health equals how well you implement all 7 Keys."

What Dr. Fuhrman is saying in his equation, however, is that for every food you could calculate a ratio of nutrients to calories. The more nutrients there are per calorie, the healthier the food choice would be. For example, if a carrot had 75 nutrients and only 10 calories, that would make it a healthier choice than a toaster pastry with 10 nutrients and 450 calories.

This equation is very important because those nutrients are the battery packs that turn on the enzymes that convert all those macro nutrients into fuel for you. When you have more fuel than furnace, you have metabolic imbalance—vitamin and mineral deficiency. Metabolic imbalance you never correct leads to metabolic diseases like diabetes.

This is exactly what happens when you eat refined sugars like common table sugar or corn syrup. Millions of dollars have been squandered on silly commercials to tell you that corn syrup is just as good for you as white sugar. Well, yes, they're both *horrible*! The plants these products originally came from contained the nutrients that would have enabled you to process the sugars, but all those nutrients have been stripped away at the factory leaving you with a lot of fuel and no micro nutrients to help you burn it.

Is it really that big a deal? Yes, it is that big a deal. It is dangerous for you and your kids. I have not bought a bag of white sugar or a bottle of corn syrup in the past decade. I have four kids who don't eat that stuff, and they aren't deprived. My seventeen-year-old son has never had a Coke®. If you offered him one, he'd turn you down cold. He's never had a "Happy Meal" either, and he'd tell you sincerely, he's a lot happier without it.

Some facts about cancer and sugar

While we're on the subject, there are two other cancer facts you should know about. First, cancer cells don't eat like other cells. They are sugar-feeders only. Second, cancer cells live in a more acid environment than normal cells. Keeping your sugar down and your pH up are two more tips for discouraging cancer growth in your body.

When your body is very acidic all over, or when you have pockets of acidity, your risk of developing cancer is much higher. In chapter 6 we will talk about the relationship between diet and acidity—how a diet rich in animal products favors disease. Acidic conditions are low-oxygen conditions and cells can't live very long in an oxygen-deprived environment without beginning fermentation.

Just how true is it that sugar is a problem? Otto Warburg is also famous for inventing the PET scan, which is still very often used to detect cancer in the body. It works by injecting the patient with radioactive *sugar* which is then traceable on the scan. This is effective for only one reason: the cancer cells grab the sugar first.

If you doubt all this, do your homework; and remember, I'm not trying to suggest "the cure" here, I'm just trying to give you some incentive to breathe better and live healthier. I don't claim to be a researcher or a cancer expert. Very few people who do research like Otto Warburg write books. They don't have time. You'll not get much information in this world first-hand or even second. It's your choice who and what you believe; always was, always will be. All of this information can be gleaned from the work of Otto Warburg mentioned above. It's readily available online.

Andi Scores—finding the nutrients

Have you ever seen tags on foods in the grocery stores telling you what "Andi" score a particular food gets? Andi scores are related to Dr. Fuhrman's health equation[4]. Nutrient density scores have actually been calculated for many common food items, and you can use this as a guide when you buy groceries. The higher the score, the better the food is for you. It's a great resource you should become familiar with.

I'll take a moment to mention that vitamins, in nature, are incredibly complicated, and that they always exist in complexes—not in isolation. While the government may adopt very narrow definitions for vitamins, these are not the same things you find in fresh fruits and veggies. Real vitamins can not be manufactured in a factory, because real vitamins can't be made out of chemicals. They may have the same formula on paper, but that's not good enough.

If your child were missing and you offered a description of him to the police, they could probably find a lot of children to match your description, but this is one instance where "close enough" just isn't good enough. You would know whether the child they found was really yours. The same is true with vitamins. Your body isn't stupid, it knows when they're the real McCoy. A paper description just doesn't do them justice.

In addition to the inadequacy of chemical formulas to fully define vitamins, there are new essential substances discovered every day—the phytonutrients. Scientists haven't even the faintest idea yet what the RDA would be for hundreds of these new discoveries and they certainly aren't in any once-daily vitamin pill.

Consider this *partial* list of known nutrients in a single ordinary beet:

3-hydroxytyramine, acetamide, aconitic acid, adenine, adipic acid, alanine, allantion, alpha-linoleic acid, alpha spinasteryl glucoside, alpha tocopherol, aluminum, arginine, arsenic, ascorbic acid, ash, aspartic acid, barium, beta carotene, beta indoleacetic acid, beta sitosterol, betaine, betanidine, betanin, betanine, boron, bromine, cadmium, caffeic acid, calcium, carbohydrates, chlorogenic acid, chromium, citric acid, cobalt, coniferin, copper, cystine, d-alpha-oxyglutaric acid, d-ribose, daucic acid, dioxymalonic acid, farnesol, fat, ferulic acid, fiber, folacin, formaldehyde, gaba, galactose, glucose, glutamic acid, glutaric acid, glycine, glycocerebroside, glyoxalic acid, guanine, guanosine, heteroxanthin, hexosans, histidine, homogentisinic acid, hydantoin, hydrocaffeic acid, hypozanthin, invertase, iron, isoleucine, kaempferol, kaempferol-glycosine, kilocalories, l-arabinose, lead, leucine, linoleic acid, lithium, lysine, magnesium, manganese, melilotic acid mercury, methionine, molybdenum mufa, neobetanin, niacin, nickel, nitrogen, oleanolic acid 3-o-beta-d-glucopyranoside, oleic acid, ornithine, oxalic acid, oxycitronic acid, p-courmaric acid, p-hydroxy-benzoic acid, palmitic acid, pantothenic acid, pentosans, phenylalanine, phosphorus, phytosterols, potassium, praebetanine, praline, protein, protoporphyrin, pufa, quercetin, quercetin-glucoside, quinic acid, raffinose, raphanol, riboflavin, rubidium, salicylic acid, sedoheptulose, selenium, serine, sfa, silicon, sodium, stearic acid, strontium, sucrose, sulfur, syringic acid, tartaric acid, thiamin, threonine, tin, titanium, tricarballyl acid, tryptophan, tyrosine, valine, vanillic acid, vanillin, vit-b-6, vulgaxanthin-I, vulgaxanthin-II, water, xylose, zinc, zirconium

One natural food beats one multivitamin, no contest.

Phytonutrient power

As you can see, plant-based diets are superior in their ability to meet human nutritional needs by virtue of the shear number of nutrients in each plant. Meat is not nearly so mysterious. If it were possible to discover new "super nutrients" in meat, those who profit from the sale of meat would definitely be exploiting that marketing strategy to its fullest potential. Yet, when was the last time you turned on the news and heard about a remarkable new nutrient with cancer-fighting potential discovered in pork chops?

It is vitally important that you not underestimate the power of fruits and veggies to enhance your health. There are so many more nutrients in them that have yet to even be named, never mind understood. One thing they nearly all seem to have in common, however, is that they all seem to be cancer fighters. With at least one in three Americans succumbing to cancer, it makes sense to eat as many as you can.

Every week it seems that somebody discovers a new "superfruit." It's nearly always available only from some place far away and is accordingly expensive to obtain. The truth is that God didn't make any junk—all fruits and veggies truly are superfoods. We just haven't learned everything about them yet. There is absolutely no need to pay extra for a mystical plant from a remote South American jungle when you have so many fresh fruits and veggies full of healing power right here at your own doorstep.

Why are plants so rich in phytonutrients, vitamins, and minerals? Plants are nothing like animals. Animals have to eat to live. Plants draw minerals and water from the soil and energy from the sun and use them to make food for animals and people. That's amazing when you think about it.

Form matters

It's also why vitamin pills don't work so well. Obviously when plants take up minerals from the soil they change them. Common sense, and labels, tell us not to go to the hardware store and eat a bag of fertilizer—even if it's organic. Those nutrients are not in the right form for us, even though they are good for plants. Plants are like little leafy processing plants, no pun intended, to make these nutrients bio-available for people and animals. You just can't walk barefoot in the garden and assimilate calcium carbonate from the mud between your toes. You aren't made to do that, and soil or rock forms of minerals, which is the carbonate form most supplements use, aren't made for you—that's plant food.

To sum up our crash course on the importance of nutrition in health:

- H = 7K, your health is based on your application of all 7 Keys to AWESOME health.

- When you don't have enough energy and building materials, you are falling apart faster than you are healing. This catabolic state leads to degenerative disease.

- Examples of degenerative disease include heart disease, diabetes, and cancer.

- Energy and building materials have to come from your diet.

- Energy comes from macro nutrients: proteins, fats, and carbohydrates.

- Energy is produced by the enzyme-driven activities within the Kreb's cycle.

- Energy can't be released from the macro-nutrients without the micro-nutrients.

- Micronutrients, sometimes called cofactors, are vitamins, minerals, and phytonutrients.

- Building materials come from the macronutrients.

- Building materials also can't be used without micro-nutrients.

- Vitamins are not all created equal. Good vitamins are made in plants, not factories.

- Nutrients (macro and micro nutrients) and calories make a ratio that determines the quality of your diet.

- Lots of nutrients, fewer calories is the path to good nutrition.

- Andi scores are a good measure to help you choose healthy food.

Now that you have some foundation in nutrition, let's really dive in and learn how to apply it.

PROVEN dietary guidelines

In this section, I'm going to give you some PROVEN dietary guidelines. I call them PROVEN partly because that just happens to be the only useful acronym these letters would spell. I find it funny, however, because if ever there were a topic you probably shouldn't apply that word to, it would be diet.

I don't think there is any more controversial, polarizing, infuriating topic in all the health care world. People can be downright hateful about it sometimes, attacking family members and friends; trying to "save" each other from nutritional heresy over the dinner table; dragging religion, politics, and family tradition through the mud in the process.

I am confident that there is nothing, absolutely nothing, I could say in this chapter that would not bring criticism and argument from at least one third of those who read it—that would be true no matter what I said! All I have to offer in my defense is that what I say here is based on what I've seen work. I've tried to offer explanations as to why it works based on what I've studied. My explanations may prove someday to be inadequate descriptions of what I've seen, but the observations remain true.

Sadly, you, too, may need to defend your choices. If you find yourself under "friendly fire," remember that studies aren't always what they seem to be. If you google "why is a meat-based diet so bad for you?" you'll find logical answers. If you google "why is a vegetarian diet so bad for you?" you'll find just as many.

Why are there hardly any studies cited in this book?

Have you ever heard two kids playing that annoying "is so—is not" game? The battle over correct nutrition comes down to nothing more than that if you rely only on so-called scientific studies.

This is why I don't include a bunch of studies and references in this book. They don't work anymore. The information age has produced a glut of research we can't wade through and don't trust anyway. We all know many results are engineered by people who were paid to achieve a desired outcome. I would rather help you think for yourself.

A major problem with scientific studies in the field of health and nutrition is that they are anything but scientific. Think about it. If I wanted to prove the PROVEN dietary guidelines, could a study actually be designed that would be accurate? The answer is no. It's not possible to study health that way. Even if I could round up a thousand people, lock them up, and feed them what I wanted to feed them, all of them would completely ruin the effect of the experiment by either hating me for taking them away from their everyday lives or thanking me for the same.

This goes back to chapter one. We can never hope to control attitude factors for 100 or more random people over the course of several months, yet attitude does influence diet and nutrition profoundly. Every person who enters a study has a different level of vitamins and minerals in reserve within their bodies. Their hormone levels are unique. They are in varying states of catabolism versus anabolism. Some are fit; others aren't. Some sleep well; others don't. All of these variables influence the outcome of the study. My point is that there are too many variables we can't control—some of them we don't even fully understand.

The futility of studying isolated nutrients

Studies on specific nutrients are pointless. What about all the other nutrients these people are getting? There are compensations in a living body. What about the health status of the people going into the study? What about food allergies? What about other stress factors?

There is *no such thing* as a "scientific" study on nutrition because the implication is that we are looking at an *isolated* variable. We *can't* isolate the variables in health! It's not possible. That's why studies are contradictory or inconclusive so much of the time. Basic knowledge of physiology, chemistry, physics, common sense, and personal experience are your best tools.

If you don't think I've got a handle on this issue, hear what legendary researcher T. Colin Campbell has to say on this subject on page 21 in his book, *The China Study*.

"I've been wrestling with public confusion for more than two decades. I can confidently state that one of the major sources of confusion is this: far too often, *we scientists focus on details while ignoring the larger context*. For example, we pin our efforts and our hopes on one isolated nutrient at a time, whether it is vitamin A to prevent cancer or vitamin E to prevent heart attacks. *We oversimplify and disregard the infinite complexity of nature.* Often, investigating minute biochemical parts of food and trying to reach broad conclusions about diet and health leads to contradictory results. Contradictory results lead to confused scientists and policy makers, and to an increasingly confused public."[7] *(Emphasis mine.)*

You can't look at everything in life through the bottom of a test tube. Too many things won't fit in there. I've heard that a Harvard medical professor once told his first-year students that 50% of what they learned in medical school would be disproved during the scope of their careers. It's no wonder—there's still so much we just don't know. I've also heard that certain high-profile medical centers are very happy when they achieve 50% accuracy in diagnosis. I'm not saying this to criticize the medical community. I'm pointing out that we're all human. It's not rational for any of us to be adamant about anything based purely on "science." Science is not sacred or infallible; it's far too easy to manipulate.

PROVEN Dietary Guidelines: the acronym for health

When you are trying to work out a really difficult problem with lots of conflicting information, it can be helpful to take it all down to the simplest, most essential level. Make a list of things you're sure of and see if that's enough to get you where you need to go. This book is the culmination of my efforts to do just that over the past twenty years. Where diet is concerned, I have distilled everything I could find and experience, and I have six guidelines to offer you. Use these 6 guidelines to make good decisions every time you get hungry. This is my PROVEN way to eat for health:

P lant-sourced food is superior to animal-sourced food.

R aw food is more healthful than cooked food.

O rganic food is superior to chemically produced food.

V ariety is critical for excellent health.

E nzymatically active food is better than dead food.

N utrient density is top priority.

Plant-sourced food is superior to animal-sourced food.

This is a hard pill for most people to swallow. In the interest of increasing profits, the giants of the meat and dairy industry have spent billions over the years to make it so. But we can not allow ourselves to be so impractical in our approach to one of the most important topics to our continued existence as to be swayed by propaganda or enslaved to tradition.

To quote T. Colin Campbell once again from page 27 of *The China Study,* "The story of protein is part science, part culture, and a good dose of mythology. The dogma surrounding protein censures, reproaches and guides, directly or indirectly, almost every thought we have in biomedical research."[7] Campbell's entire career has focused on protein research, so he ought to know.

The reasons I say that a plant-based diet is superior to an animal-based diet centers around the following issues:

1. The design of the human digestive tract.

2. The relative ability of each to meet human needs.

3. The relative dangers each present to the human population.

Let's look at each of the more closely.

1. Digestive Design

We have already discussed the design of the human digestive system in chapter 3. Just as a recap, we were made with flat molars ill-suited to the handling of meat but ideal for grinding grains, fruits, and veggies. We have insufficient stomach acid to safely handle meat. We have a long and winding intestinal tract which is easily obstructed by fiberless food (meat). The length of our intestine is like that of animals known to be primarily or entirely plant-eaters.

When humans eat meat, the process of digestion is slowed down, and the transit time is such that meat rots before we can excrete it. This rotting pollutes the intestinal tract with all sorts of toxic, acidic by-products which are absorbed into the blood stream and circulated through our tissues, raising the potential for pH disturbances either systemically or locally, which increases our risk for degenerative disease.

2. Meeting human nutritional needs

At this time, we don't know precisely what is required to keep a human healthy for a lifetime. We have the RDA, which is our official best guess, but we know it to be grossly inadequate. It takes an awful lot of testing before the government is willing to go out on a limb and say that a certain quantity of a vitamin is the necessary minimum for health. This has been done for only a small fraction of the known micronutrients, and we are discovering new ones every year.

The RDA is meant to establish the *minimum* required amount, with occasionally a little extra margin for safety, for each nutrient to prevent overt disease—not the optimal amount for vibrant health. Each person is biochemically unique. That means that while 145 micrograms of iodine daily might be enough to prevent a visible goiter for me, it might not be for you.

The inter-play between the nutrients goes so far as to include substitutions and conversions in the body. There is no way to truly ever establish one right combination of minimums that will keep all people well.

The PROVEN guidelines are designed to take all of these factors into account. Plant-based diets honor the design of the human digestive system while meaty diets clog the works both at the intestinal level and at the cellular level by increasing the toxic/acidic load in the body.

Human nature is a funny thing. As long as you are doing what everybody else is doing, nobody worries what you're grazing on, but as soon as one antelope breaks from the herd, all the other heads go up. Everybody gets excited and starts asking questions and raising safety concerns. So let's address a couple of common fears before moving on. The biggest concerns are always protein and calcium.

3. Dangers. What about protein and calcium?

We discussed protein in chapter 3. For a quick review, there is no shortage of protein in a plant-based diet. The larger animals people usually want to eat got their protein needs met by eating plants, and they have more muscle and bone than any human being. Think of the biggest animals on the planet—elephants, giraffes, and draft horses. They have very large bones and huge muscles, all built from eating grasses, grains, and leaves. Besides all that, the human body recycles 80% of its proteins, so your daily need is quite small.

The very same argument holds true for the calcium issue. We've been sold out by industry and agency to believe we need massive amounts of calcium to prevent osteoporosis and that it should come from dairy sources. Both beliefs are false.

If you search statistically for which countries have the highest intakes of dairy and which countries have the highest rates of osteoporosis, you find they are the same countries. High dairy calcium intake does absolutely nothing to protect you from osteoporosis; on the contrary, it is a diet high in meat and dairy that aggravates it by causing acidity in the blood which robs the bones of calcium and slows the body's healing. By contrast, in some cultures, such as many parts of rural Asia, people consume no dairy and eat precious little or no meat at all and osteoporosis is virtually unheard of among them.

If you want to prove this for yourself, grab a turkey and take out the wishbone. Drop it, the bone not the turkey, into a glass of cheap white vinegar and leave it for a day or two. When you take it out, find a friend and make a wish. (Try to break it.) You'll find it intriguingly flexible. That's because vinegar is highly acidic and the acid pulls the calcium out of the bone. Now try breaking a piece of chalk. Brittle, right? Chalk is almost pure calcium.

When there is a lack of calcium, bones bend, they don't break. I don't need a forty-million-dollar study to figure out that calcium deficiency is not the whole story behind osteoporosis.

Healthy bone is built on a healthy protein matrix. Ever heard the expression "bouncing baby boy?" Babies' bones are notoriously resilient; they seldom break. When a baby is born, its bones are not calcified yet. They are almost entirely collagen; that's the protein matrix. Over time, due to the stresses of weight-bearing exercise, those rubbery little bones collect calcium and other minerals to become hardened so they will support the child's larger frame.

When adults' bones become brittle, most of the fault lies with that protein matrix. Due to hormonal imbalances, poor diet, poor digestion, lack of exercise, and ill-advised use of antacids, the protein matrix degrades to the point that it can't hold calcium and other minerals effectively. The result is brittle bone in which cells are dying faster than they can be replaced.

There is an inverse relationship between acids in your stomach and minerals and proteins in your system. Without sufficient acid in your stomach, you can't properly absorb minerals and break down proteins. Good digestion is your first-line defense against osteoporosis.

Osteoporosis drugs destroy your body's ability to get rid of old dead bone cells. This is why your test results indicate an increase in density—you're still making some new cells, but the old ones are still there also. Your increased density is made, increasingly, of dead tissue. This is why they warn you about checking out jaw pain while taking these drugs. Some people develop a necrotic infection as a direct result of carrying around dead bone tissue. It's also why the risk of fracture actually goes up once you've been on the drugs for several years.

By now, meat enthusiasts are surely considering the old arguments about complete protein. Even the Center for Disease Control (CDC) has abandoned the idea that complete protein is important, but in case you're unfamiliar with the theory… Meat, it is often said, contains all the essential amino acids in one place while almost no plants do. You supposedly need meat so that you can enjoy "one-stop shopping" for all your amino acid needs.

Why do we care so much about getting all our amino acids in one food? How come no one talks about vitamin-complete food where all the known RDA vitamins are contained in one food? Because we all know it doesn't matter. It is no more useful or necessary to get all your amino acids in one food than it is to get all your vitamins or minerals in one food. Are you really only going to eat one food? If you did, should it be a plant or a meat? Where would you get the most nutrients? Hmmmm……

As for protein quantity, you really don't need much. Some people believe that you need a lot of protein to be "strong." There is no advantage to exceeding your requirement for any macronutrient; in fact, it's quite the opposite. It is common knowledge that exceeding your requirement for carbs is bad—leads to excess weight and diabetes. Excess fat is condemned by the cardio world—not good for the cardiovascular system. Why do we think that excess protein is the exception where more is going to be better?

Excess protein creates excess acids in your body which contribute to every kind of disease. We don't know everything about the dangers of excess protein, but the culmination of T. Colin Campbell's research—not lab studies only, but mountains of demographic evidence from millions of real people in real life—included the following findings: cancer only grew when the amount of dietary protein intake "exceeded the amount of dietary protein needed to satisfy their body growth rate." Even more interesting news: "plant protein did *not* promote cancer growth, even at the higher levels of intake."

What constitutes excess protein in humans? The RDA for protein varies with age and gender. Figure 1 on the next page is a chart found on the CDC's official website: (www.cdc.gov/nutrition/everyone/basics/protein.htm).

Figure 1. RDA for Protein

Recommended Daily Allowance for Protein	
	Grams of protein needed each day
Children ages 1–3	13
Children ages 4–8	19
Children ages 9–13	34
Girls ages 14–18	46
Boys ages 14–18	52
Women ages 19–70+	46
Men ages 19–70+	56

Source: Center for Disease Control

How can you know how much is really enough? Consider this test case. Because of their high growth rate, babies arguably need more protein during their first year of life than they ever will again. No one debates that the perfect food for a human baby is human milk. Human milk is not more than 5% protein. The U.S. RDA is 10% or more. What the math says is that half the RDA is more than enough for an adult. The real adult need for protein is amply met by about 30g daily. To give you perspective, 30g of protein is about the weight of ten pennies.

Most of the current misconception about the need for large amounts of protein is based on studies done more than 75 years ago. In these studies it was found that rats needed a large amount of protein. Rats and humans are radically different. Rat milk, for example is 45% protein, while human milk is only 5% protein. Based on these facts, it seems very safe to say that humans and rats have radically different protein requirements and we need to adjust our thinking about the role of protein in human nutrition.

There is protein in every whole food—no exceptions. It's extremely easy to get the RDA of protein. Too easy. If you ate a small bowl of oatmeal and a cluster of grapes for breakfast, you'd be eating about 7g of protein. If you had a salad with sunflower seeds and a little dried fruit on it with a bowl of vegetable soup for lunch, you'd be getting about 22g of protein. A granola bar snack in the afternoon could provide another 10g of protein. Brown rice with stir-fried veggies for dinner would give you another 15g of protein. Your total for the day would be about 54g. You've already exceeded your real need—almost twice, without a single bite of meat.

I've mentioned Campbell a lot. Do other well-known doctors with proven track records agree that plant-based nutrition is superior to animal? Ornish, Esselstyn, McDougall, Klapper, Fuhrman, Barnard, the entire membership

(125,000+) of the Physician's Committee for Responsible Medicine, how many would you like? For more information see http://pcrm.org.

Every organization from the American Cancer Society to the American Heart Association and others all acknowledge that fruits and vegetables offer protection from the diseases they are trying to cure. The USDA has always acknowledged the critical role of fruits and vegetables in human health, and their suggestions for intake have increased steadily with each new official recommendation from the old four food groups to the more modern pyramid and now the plate diagram.

Again, will one steak kill you? Of course not. The human body is amazingly adaptable and complex with all sorts of compensation ability and back-up systems. We were designed for survival. Yes, you have the ability to eat a piece of meat and live to tell about it. That's not the question. We're talking about what's good for you, what will help you live longer in good health, what will help you thrive—not just survive.

No food is neutral

Though the damage or the benefit varies significantly from one food to another, no food is neutral. It helps or it hurts. One piece of meat, one chunk of cheese, one piece of cake, or one cookie—they're all negatives to some degree, no matter where they came from. Every one of them causes damage on some level and moves you away from your health goals. One apple, one spear of broccoli, one almond, one small green salad—they're all positives that help you get where you want to go.

You can repair the damage bad foods cause, but it's a drain on your body's resources that will eventually take its toll on your quality and length of life. You can not cheat the system without paying the price. The sicker you are already, the higher the price in the near future.

I can take just so many bites of food in one day. I'm not going to waste many of them on a nutritional investment that doesn't pay good dividends, whether it's steak or cheesecake. That's the bottom line. Why do we think of junky food as a treat anyway?

Raw food is superior to cooked food

It was discovered long ago that when you cook food, you alter the structure of the proteins, sugars, and fats in the food. You don't need scientists for this one either, just cook an egg in a hot skillet and see if it looks the same as when it came out of the shell. The changes you observe are largely changes to the proteins in the egg.

Proteins are long chains of amino acids. The exact sequence of amino acids tells you what sort of protein you're looking at and its shape largely defines its function. You can get a mental picture of proteins by picturing the amino acids as a child's string of plastic pop beads. These are large plastic beads with a hole on one end and a nub on the other. They pop together easily to form long flexible chains. You can twist the chains into all sorts of interesting shapes. If you take a blow torch to one of these pop-bead chains, the plastic will melt and the shape of your creation will be lost. The beads obviously won't function the way they did before.

Damage to proteins can be superficial or very deep. If it goes so far as to damage the amino acids themselves, you won't benefit nutritionally from the food at all. Low heat may allow you obtain many of the nutrients in a cooked food, but no one really cooks food at temperatures low enough to prevent significant damage. You can part out an old car, but not after you incinerate it. The longer you cook meat or any other food, and the higher the temperature, the more damaged the proteins and other nutrients are.

Keep in mind that your body does not use the protein you eat "as is." You take it apart and use the amino acids to build the proteins you need. Your ability to make enough proteins to build your own healthy cells depends not just on how much protein you take in, but also on how much of it is still usable, and how well you can break it down. If you can't take it apart and use it, you have to excrete it, which is a burden on your liver and kidneys. Your ability to digest protein is a key factor here. Most people who have a "protein deficiency" are eating plenty of protein, but they are not digesting and absorbing it. Eating more protein that you can't digest anyway won't fix that problem.

The most vital site of protein digestion is the stomach. Acid is produced in your stomach to denature the complex proteins you eat so that enzymes in your stomach and intestines can disassemble the long chains of amino acids. If you can't break them down, or they are too damaged to be useful, what happens to them? They pass on into your intestine where they may cause irritation. If there is irritation or damage already, they may pass on into your bloodstream. In your bloodstream, a foreign protein is treated as a serious threat. Your immune system declares war and creates an antibody army to attack the invader.

In 1930, Dr. Paul Kautchakoff discovered this effect. (http://www.healthe-livingnews.com/articles/are_enzyme-deficient_foods_making_you_sick.html) He showed that eating cooked and processed foods produces a condition in the body called digestive leukocytosis. That's a big term for white blood cells rushing to defend you against unhealthy food. When your immune system is preoccupied with attacking your food, it can't concentrate all its energy on killing bad bacteria and viruses and keeping you well. It begins, even in healthy people, when you cross the 50 yard line on the raw food field—meaning more than 50% of your food is cooked.

In less healthy individuals, or those with compromised immune systems, the ability to tolerate cooked food can be much lower. Some people can not tolerate any cooked food at all without triggering massive autoimmune reaction. Fibromyalgia and lupus sufferers take note.

The bottom line here, is that eating cooked food, no matter how healthy you are, increases the level of immune system stimulation and inflammation everywhere in your body. No pill can suspend the effects of gravity for you, and swallowing anti-inflammatories like candy or killing your immune system with chemotherapy will never stop digestive leukocytosis.

If cooked food were superior to raw, or even equally acceptable, why would your body attack it? The human body is well-equipped with acids to denature proteins, emulsifiers to break up fats, and enzymes to digest all three macro-nutrients. Why would we need to cook the food to "help" the process along?

How are fats and sugars affected by heat? When fats get too hot, they hydrogenate and so are prevented from functioning as they should in your body. Starches, and therefore sugars, become more concentrated through cooking. If you ate raw sweet potatoes, you would probably not want even one whole sweet potato of modest size. When you cook them, you find that you want to eat three times as much. This has implications for weight control and blood sugar control, both of which respond very well to increasing the amount of raw vegetables in your diet.

Another problem with cooking food is the formation of cancer-causing substances that occurs at temperatures lower than those at which we usually cook. A classic example is acrylamide, a carcinogen that is formed in starchy foods, such as French fries, when they are heated beyond 248°F. French fries are the only vegetable some children ever eat these days; what does that say about the state of children's health in this country? When was the last time you ate anything cooked at less than 248°F? Here's a clue: when any food begins to brown, you've already created a multitude of carcinogens.

Because there are several different kinds of "sensors" in your stomach to tell you when you've had enough to eat, raw food satisfies in a healthier way. Some sensors detect the richness of food, others detect the degree to which your stomach stretches. A few bites of rich food might satisfy the richness receptors, and they also might supply all the calories you need; but the stretch receptors are not appeased and your nutrient needs are not met.

Raw foods, on the other hand, can make all the difference, giving you the feeling of fullness and the satisfaction of meeting your nutrient needs without adding more calories than you can ever burn. Some raw foods, such as coconut and avocado, can even meet the demands of the richness receptors.

It has long been claimed that on some level, cooked food is actually easier to digest than raw food—the opposite of what I suggest here. The benefit of cooking, is that the break-down process is partially accomplished by cooking so you don't have to do all the work. I even read one author who claimed that the act of chewing required too much loss of energy, so cooked food was clearly better. I have two comments about that theory.

One is that chewing processes food quite well if you do it thoroughly. Thorough chewing, plus the plant enzymes and salivary enzymes, makes nutrients bound by indigestible substances like cellulose available to you just as cooking would. Additionally, I see it as painfully obvious that the author never did his own cooking, otherwise he would have known that chewing takes a lot less energy than meal preparation ever did.

It has long been common knowledge that some nutrient content is lost through cooking. Vitamins and minerals can be destroyed or removed by cooking. While a few micronutrients appear to become more bioavailable through cooking, and most people do not need to eat all their food raw, there is no doubt that eating a high percentage of raw food can only be beneficial to your health.

Organic food is superior to non-organic food

Although there are still a few die-hards out there who say that chemically produced food is equivalent to organic in every way that matters, I don't think anyone takes them seriously anymore. To suggest that carcinogenic pesticide residue is harmless is an idea that anyone with half a grain of common sense can dismiss without any help from me.

There is more to the concept of organic produce than simply the absence of pesticide—it's a completely different agricultural philosophy. You might say organic agriculture is to plants as natural health is to humans. It's all about working with nature to make the plant as healthy as possible by meeting all of its needs abundantly, and without chemicals.

Because of this philosophy, organic produce has the potential to be nutritionally superior to non-organic because of the nutrient density of the soil it was grown in. If you think about it logically, no plant is any better than the soil it grew in. If that soil is deficient, the plant will be also. Healthy soil is not possible when there is heavy chemical use. Artificial vitamins and minerals are no better for a plant than they are for a human.

Healthy soil is a complex study all by itself. You could walk onto most farms and determine for yourself how healthy the soil is. There are several things to look for: the first sign of healthy soil is that it should be loose and fairly uniform. Dry, cracked soil in large chunks is clearly not ideal. The soil should also be a rich dark color. There should be bits and pieces of decaying plant material mixed in with the dirt, and there should be worms. Lots and lots of worms.

Healthy worms are one of the best indicators of healthy soil. They are not only there because the soil is healthy; they also help to make it healthy by eating the decaying plant matter and excreting the waste. It sounds gross, but it's a very effective way to improve soil quality. Along with a healthy worm population, there should be a healthy population of good soil bacteria to further break down decaying plant matter.

Sadly, due to the excessive use of chemicals on American farmland—which is only made worse by the spread of GMO crops—there are now many farms with so little life left in the soil that the waste from last year's crop won't even decay when you till it under. If the soil won't even support microbial and vermicular life, how well do think it will support human life?

On an organic farm, if you fail to properly prepare the soil, your plants will not grow well, and you can't just dump chemicals on them to compensate. If your plants aren't healthy, they will be attacked by insects, and you can't obliterate them with pesticides to compensate. On an organic farm, it's a lot harder to fake it.

I could say that studies have shown organic produce to be higher in nutrients than non-organic, but you could find others that would say otherwise. They don't always compare things fairly.

One reason studies sometimes find no difference between organic and non-organic produce has to do with supply and demand. Because the public does not buy (demand) more organic produce, the supply chain is not as efficient. Organic produce may take longer to reach your local store, and it may stay there longer than conventional produce. These delays reduce the nutritional value of the food.

I have done my own "research" and found that there is a very big difference in the way organic and non-organic produce tastes and behaves. If you are into fresh juice as I am, you may have seen the difference in organic versus non-organic carrot juice firsthand. When I juice non-organic carrots, the first thing I notice is that I can't stand the taste. The second is that it doesn't look the same. Non-organic juice separates more rapidly with a little bright orange material settling to the bottom and a lot of dingy brown watery stuff at the top. The consistency, even when it's not separated, is very thin and watery, while organic juice is thicker, and there is often an oily sheen at the top.

Is non-organic any good? Certainly there is nutritional value in non-organic produce, and you can definitely get healthier eating it; but again, we aren't talking about surviving, we're talking about thriving, and there is a lot of evidence that organic can be superior.

The solution to this problem is two-fold. First you have to be selective. Buying organic isn't always the best choice. I'll buy a conventional pear that looks perfect long before I'll buy a moldy, shriveled organic one. Second, it's a good idea to try to buy local produce when you can. It may mean an extra trip here and there, but it's well worth the effort. The added nutritional value of locally-grown non-organic produce may be higher than organic produce improperly picked and shipped from far away.

To help you decide when to buy organic, here's a list prepared by the Environmental Working Group (www.ewg.org). These are foods often referred to as the dirty dozen because they are known to have the highest levels of pesticides, making it more important to look for organically grown produce.

12 Most Contaminated Foods

• Peaches	• Apples
• Sweet Bell Peppers	• Celery
• Nectarines	• Strawberries
• Cherries	• Pears
• Grapes (Imported)	• Spinach
• Lettuce	• Potatoes

Notice that when grapes are listed it says "imported." This is because American produce is typically less dangerous than produce grown in third world countries. We have the nasty habit of banning extremely hazardous chemicals here, then selling them to third-world farmers who treat their crops and sell the contaminated produce back to us. It's something you want to be aware of. Really, it should be illegal to sell those chemicals anywhere.

To round out this section, here's a list of the least contaminated foods that are relatively safe to buy non-organically. Organic is still superior when it's fresh, but when availability is poor and money is tight, we need to make the best choices we can.

12 Least Contaminated

- Onions
- Sweet Corn (Frozen)
- Mango
- Sweet Peas (Frozen)
- Bananas
- Broccoli
- Avocado
- Pineapples
- Asparagus
- Kiwi Fruit
- Cabbage
- Papaya

Since we don't know the sum total of all human nutritional needs, and we may never know, it's best to eat a wide variety of fresh foods. Remember the page of nutrients that can be found in an ordinary beet? It's incredible. A similar list could be made for any fruit or vegetable—they're all that complex. That's why every fruit or vegetable is a superfood.

For optimal health you need to take on the "no vegetable left behind" challenge. Learn at least one way to prepare every vegetable you can find in your local stores. If you really don't like something, you don't have to keep eating it, but you'll probably be able to expand your list of things you like significantly. Each time you shop, bring home one thing you've never had before and look around to see just how many types of produce you've never eaten. It might surprise you how big a rut you're in.

Most people don't realize how limited their food selection really is. To test yours, write down everything you eat for a week. At the end of the week, review your record and list all the different foods you ate. It might be a pretty short list. If there are fewer than 35 items, you have a very limited diet.

In a typical week I would have a list similar to this:

Lettuce	Blueberries	Celery
Tomatoes	Strawberries	Garlic
Carrots	Raspberries	Whole grain bread
Onions	Blackberries	Millet
Apples	Almonds	Sweet potatoes
Brown rice	Grapefruit	Cashews
Bananas	Oranges	Pecans
Kiwi	Spinach	Sunflower seeds
Avocados	Plums	White potatoes
Coconut	Green beans	Peas
Black beans	Navy beans	Great northern beans
Cucumbers	Olives	Garbanzo beans
Cranberries	Raisins	Beets
Broccoli	Cauliflower	Black-eyed peas
Kale	Pineapple	Cantaloupe
Eggplant	Kidney beans	Brussels sprouts
Bell peppers	Asparagus	There's more...

Yes, I really do eat these things in a typical week. So does the rest of my family—even the children. I have kids who get genuinely excited by the sight of a really excellent salad bar, and they love to make and drink fresh juice.

Enzyme-rich food is superior to dead food

This is another idea that seems to spark debate in certain circles. It's because it "can't be scientifically proven" that enzymes can confer health benefits to you when you eat them. Or can it?

If you're scientifically inclined, consider the laws of thermodynamics. These are natural laws accepted by the scientific community about how matter and energy behave in the universe. According to the rules, energy can not be created and it can not be destroyed. If enzymes are capable of doing work, and they definitely are when they are "alive," then they also have energy.

Where does that energy go when you eat them? What effect does that energy have?

Everything in the universe has its own frequency. All matter vibrates constantly. This is not controversial at all. Every organ in your body has a frequency. Food has frequency. Every molecule has frequency. Frequencies change when an organ isn't healthy or a food is cooked—dead. For example, the frequency of a cancerous tumor is low, about 30 MHz.

Figure 2. Food frequencies[16]

Foods and Organs	MHz
Hamburger	5
Cake	1—3
Synthetic vitamins	10 - 30
Raw Almonds	40 - 50
Green Vegetables	70 - 90
Normal liver	55 - 60
Normal colon	58 - 63
Normal stomach	58 - 65
Normal brain	72 - 78

Healthy tissues have frequencies from 55—80 MHz. Not surprisingly, healthy foods have higher frequencies than unhealthy foods. Figure 2. on the previous page will help you compare some frequencies.

What's the difference between the healthy and the unhealthy? Is it all about enzymes? Surely not; but because enzymes have frequency, they must contribute to the higher frequency of healthy foods. Can it really be pure coincidence that the healthiest foods have frequencies within the same range as healthy tissues? It is through frequencies that all things in the body operate on the most fundamental level. Frequency is a form of energy, and it can't be destroyed, but it can affect your body based on what you eat. In chemistry and physics things are attracted, or not, based on frequency. I want to eat things that won't challenge my healthy frequencies.

Studies conflict and confuse. Don't just read science. Do science. You can test these things for yourself and, at least for now, you don't need anybody's permission to try it and think it through.

Remember that enzymes are like little robotic workers that take things apart or put things together. They have their micronutrient battery packs on in fresh food, but in spoiled food, the batteries are running low. In cooked food, the battery packs are completely dead, and the enzymes are permanently deactivated.

Though cooked food enthusiasts vehemently disagree, many advocates for raw and "live" food will tell you that these live enzymes help you digest your food. They say that when you eat "dead" food with no enzymes, your body has to provide the enzymes to break down the food out of your own finite reserves. This robs your body of energy that could be used for other things— like living longer, healing, and doing work.

They also say that the amount of energy it takes for you to generate the power to digest three cooked meals each day is equivalent to the amount of energy you would use to do eight hours of strenuous physical labor. I agree with them.

The amount of energy used in digestion is huge, and there are practical ways to verify these things to some extent. If you eat an all-raw meal, you will find that you are hungry again fairly soon. Why is that? It's not because your meal was nutritionally inadequate, and it's not because you didn't eat much. It's because raw foods are less concentrated, and they digest more easily and quickly. Is this because of their enzyme content? Does it matter? You can't separate the fact that food is raw from the fact that it contains live enzymes. If you have one, you have the other.

If you eat all raw until lunchtime, you will probably find that your usual 3:00 slump doesn't happen. Why? Is it the enzymes? What we care about is what works. If you want more energy to do what you want to do, what you need is more nutrient-dense raw food. What happens to people who eat 50%, or even 85%, raw? Without exception, if they are getting a good variety, they have a lot more energy.

When you eat a meal that makes you want to sleep it off, you can bet there weren't any enzymes in it. Let's try one more experiment. Can you think of a meal that usually zonks you out? Next time you eat that, try taking 2 or 3 digestive enzyme capsules from your local health food store just before you start eating. See how you feel. Does it still knock you out, or do you have more energy and feel less heavy in the gut than you usually do? I'll bet you feel a whole lot better. This is all the proof I need that enzymes *do* make a big difference.

This is also a good tip for managing the cooked portion of your diet. Taking supplemental enzymes is a good way to help your body process cooked food without so much wear and tear and without slowing you down.

As far as proving that enzymes will extend your lifespan potential, I can't prove that, either, but I can think logically about it. No matter how much maintenance I perform on it, my car will wear out when I put enough miles on it. The more you use a physical object, the sooner it wears out and breaks down. Eating food without enzymes puts more miles on your body than eating food with enzymes. That just makes sense.

What foods are the richest sources of enzymes? Newly sprouted plants are the richest sources of enzymes, and certainly sprouts of all kinds are nutrient and enzyme dense. They also tend to be very high in protein, so we don't need too many of them. All fresh fruits and veggies, however are good sources of enzymes.

Nuts and seeds, on the other hand, are not always good sources of active enzymes. These otherwise nutritionally dense foods have some built-in defense mechanisms that make them enzyme-unfriendly unless you handle them correctly. Nuts and seeds are meant to become plants some day, and they would sprout very quickly when they fell to the ground if it were not for the enzyme-inhibitors they carry.

Enzyme inhibitors are exactly what they sound like. Enzymes are responsible for the germination process that makes a seed sprout and grow. Inhibitors don't allow that process to happen until the time is right. Soaking nuts or seeds in water for several hours tells them the time is right. Soaking unlocks the enzyme potential in the nut and makes it far easier to digest. Now that the enzymes are working for you, the nut also tastes better and it isn't quite so hard.

Every food in a bottle, can, or package of any kind has had its enzymes killed. Pasteurizing milk or juice kills enzymes; that's partly how it preserves the food so that it can be transported and stored for longer periods of time. This is also one reason a juice machine is a great investment.

Fresh juice is radically different from bottled juice you buy in the store. It has its enzymes intact and its full complement of vitamins and minerals, and it tastes better than you can imagine.

Nutrient density is top priority

Much of the information that applies to this principle has already been discussed in the preceding sections because all of this is so interrelated. Here's a review of a few pertinent facts about what nutrient density is and why it's so important:

- Nutrient density is a measure of micronutrients, not macronutrients.
- Micronutrients are vitamins, minerals, and phytonutrients.
- Macronutrients are proteins, fats, and carbohydrates.
- Nutrient density refers to the quantity of micronutrients relative to the number of calories in food.
- Micronutrients are necessary to drive the Kreb's cycle which produces energy for living, healing, and working.
- Micronutrients are the battery packs for the enzymes that facilitate all the work in the body.
- Micronutrients are largely responsible for the amount of energy your body is able to produce.

When you are shopping for food, you need to know how to quickly locate nutrient-dense food. Here are three rules to shop by:

1. Nutrient-dense food lives in the produce section and, to a slightly lesser extent, the frozen food section of your supermarket. If you visit any other aisle, you are in the dead zone.
2. Shop by color. The most brightly colored fruits and veggies usually have the most nutrients per calorie to offer you.
3. Andi scores are a reliable measurement of nutrient density.

When you combine the principle of nutrient density with the principle of variety, you have a truly powerful one-two punch against malnutrition and disease. What you choose to eat determines what materials you have to run on and to build new tissue with. It's a very important decision.

Nutrient density is the common factor in all six PROVEN guidelines. Plant foods are more nutrient dense than animal foods. Raw foods offer better nutritional value than cooked foods. Organic foods usually have higher nutrient density than chemically grown produce. Variety insures your aggregate nutrient density across the spectrum of your entire diet, and enzyme activity in your food increases your access to nutrients and your benefit from them.

As you may have realized, I call these the PROVEN dietary guidelines because I have tried to give you the means mentally and sometimes even physically, to test and prove them for yourself. As long as you are dependent on the latest study, you will never have peace or confidence in what you're doing. You will continue to be stressed by diet.

I said at the beginning that my goal was to eliminate the stress of figuring out what was right with regard to diet. That's a critical milestone in your journey to awesome health because managing your stress factors is absolutely essential to the process of healing. It's part of the A in AWESOME.

I firmly believe that if you consistently apply all six of the PROVEN guidelines yourself for at least three months, you will agree, they're PROVEN fact.

Chapter 6: Part 2

The Food Section

When I first began to learn about diet myself, I realized immediately what was missing in the world—an easy way to eat well. Everything I read was so complicated and every recipe involved so many weird ingredients I'd never heard of and couldn't get locally that I was quickly discouraged.

My criteria for good healthy food is as follows:

- It has to taste good.
- It can't be too expensive.
- It has to be made of stuff I understand—and can find.

- It can't require me to look stuff up and follow specific recipes every time I want to eat something.

- It can't take more than 20 minutes of hands-on preparation, preferably a lot less.

- It has to be something my kids can eat, too, 'cause I ain't cookin' twice!

I'm not putting anything in this book that doesn't meet those criteria. Healthy food lovers, rejoice! This is a not a diet plan or a recipe book, it's a system of thinking about food that's made to make figuring out what to eat next easy.

What should I eat? How people make choices

So, what should I eat? The eternal question… When people think about what to eat they usually do so in one of three ways:

1. What would taste good right now,

2. What's handy, or

3. What their current fad diet dictates

Food manufacturers focus on that first scenario very heavily. They make everything taste good with no true regard for your health. They use an array of flavor-enhancing chemicals to twang your buds and convince you that what you're eating tastes good even when it really doesn't. Still, some people believe the corporate giants wouldn't or couldn't sell stuff that was really bad for you. We have to wake up—healthy people aren't that gullible.

Fast food restaurants focus on the second group. They're always nearby when you're hungry, but they aren't looking out for your health at all. They are as bad about foisting 4F foods on the public as the processed food giants.

The fad-diet crowd is, at least, eating with purpose. The problem with a fad diet is that it can't last forever—and neither can the results you achieve while you're on it. Also, most fad diets are so restrictive and narrow they are truly dangerous long-term.

In anything you try, your outcome is a direct result of what you're doing, so you need a program you can stay with for life—one that DOES look out for your health, not just your weight. Can we do that? Absolutely!

Sometimes the biggest hindrance to making a diet change is concept itself. Nobody likes the idea of being "on a diet." but the word "diet" just means the stuff you usually eat. Everybody's on a diet of some sort! The concept of "diet" has been hijacked in recent years to mean that we're going to do something different—temporarily.

Who wants to be healthy temporarily? We live in a cause-and-effect world. Results last only as long as you keep doing what produces them. Your car moves forward only as long as you keep your foot on the gas. Your health will improve or hold steady only as long as you keep tending to it.

What we need is permanent change that makes our life better. The second biggest problem is that the diet concept carries with it the idea of someone else telling us what to do. Right away, we feel resistance.

This chapter will give you a new way to think about healthy eating that keeps you firmly in the driver's seat. You design your own healthy eating plan around your own tastes with as much or as little planning as you want. Spontaneity is still an option.

Managing your food psychology—a new way to think about food

If we can learn anything from big food manufacturers, it's how to manage human psychology. When you get hungry, you aren't very creative or philosophical, and the food sellers really step up to the plate with fully formed pre-packaged food ideas. Ideas are the key to their success.

Have you ever looked into a fridge or pantry full of food and said, "There's nothing to eat here!" That's the core issue for most people when they try to improve their diet—they don't have any ideas! It's all about how it's marketed to your mind.

It's easy when you go to a restaurant. You see ideas on the menu—not an inventory of ingredients. If restaurants started telling us what was in the kitchen and asking us what we wanted them to do with it no one would ever eat out again! We need a whole new paradigm to relate to our food. One that can make natural food work for us.

That's what this chapter is about—giving you a new way to categorize your natural food options so you always know what's to eat. Instead of saying tomatoes, cucumbers, lettuce, beans, etc., you need real food words.

We're going to focus on the 6 pillars of AWESOME nutrition, and here they are—in real food words: salads, smoothies and fresh fruits, soups, juices, healthy starches, and steamed vegetables. These are frameworks you can plug whatever ingredients you have into and make it work. We'll talk about precisely how to do this—methods, not just recipes; how to stock your kitchen, and what equipment you really need.

In this chapter you'll learn how to eat well at home, in restaurants, and on the road. We'll also talk about how to live your new lifestyle harmoniously with your less enthusiastic family members, and finally I'll give you some tips on how to get your kids to eat healthy, too, at every age.

Living with non-believers

Let's face it, this is a journey not everyone is ready for. If you care about your loved ones, the best thing you can give them is a stellar example, not a good talking-to! There is another natural law at work here, one that physics can't fully describe. It's the law of attraction and resistance.

When you want someone to change, they resist; when you display something desirable, they pursue it. It's basically the old Tom Sawyer principle. If you get healthy, I mean really make a big difference, at least some of the people who see it will want to get in on it. Some, not all.

You also have to be able to accept the fact that everybody has rights. If you demand your right to change, you have to respect their right not to. It's really hard, but the last thing you want to do is ruin a relationship. Stay put and stay positive because when bad health strikes, you'll be in the right place at the right time to offer real help—which they still may reject.

On a practical level, life with unhealthy eaters can be challenging. If you're a woman whose husband and children won't change, you have to deal with how to cook for them while avoiding the temptation and discouragement that come from feeling left out. There may even be comments…

If you're a man whose wife won't help you eat healthy, you may have it just as bad. Some women, wonderful wives really, are so determined to protect you from your own insanity that they can just about starve you into submission. They control the shopping and the cooking, so you have a really hard way to go. They also can be relentless with their "concern" for your well-being.

Both scenarios need specific help. So, here goes. Ladies first.

If you are a woman, you have three options. Which one is best is something only you can determine based on your family culture and values.

1. Option one: Not recommended.

Make entirely separate meals for you and for them. I mention this only because it is the most commonly attempted solution, and I want to spare you the pain of trying it. This is bad on several levels.

First, the work load alone will be discouraging, but the emotional strain of separateness you feel will crush you as a wife and mother. This messes up the attitude/stress handling aspect of the 7 Key program so bad that you probably won't succeed long term with this option.

2. Option two: This one is usually best.

Say little about it unless you're asked. Fix 75% of each meal to suit your needs and 25% to suit theirs. Let's say that before reading this book you were in the habit of fixing some sort of meat entrée along with two veggies for your family's evening meal. You can begin a transitional process wherein you fix three veggies (or two veggies and starch) in a more healthful fashion than before and you still cook the meat.

You all eat 75% of the same food at dinner so you don't stand out like a sore thumb and nobody feels so isolated. Nothing much changes for your family, except for the improved quality of the veggies and starches. No one has to give anything up. You may choose to skip the meat all or some of the time or eat a greatly reduced portion. You may have an entirely meatless meal one or more nights each week. You might also begin to slowly introduce more raw dishes—always making sure there is enough familiar fare to keep anyone from going hungry.

3. Option three: Cold, cold turkey.

This option is not for the faint of heart. You can just say, "I'm in charge of the food prep in this house, and I'm making some changes for the sake of our health. I will be happy to provide amply for all your dietary needs. If you don't like what I fix, you have my permission to learn how to cook, just be sure to clean up after yourself." This one needs no further explanation. It stands to reason that certain demographics may occasionally go to bed a bit hungry. There is more on that in the section on transitioning children.

Now for the men. More and more men are sharing equally in the household chores these days. If you are one who does, kudos to you. All the things I said to the women may apply to you also at least to some extent.

For those who live in a more traditional home setting where the wife is the head of the kitchen, well, you're in a pickle. Nevertheless, you can handle this like any other business, military, or sports situation. Grab your bootstraps—a man's gotta do what a man's gotta do, and you gotta learn to cook.

Your first step may be to very kindly explain to your wife, who loves you very much please remember, that you've made a decision and it's final. Your mind is made up and you would appreciate her support. This advice is good for the women, too.

Standing your ground is critical regardless of gender, and you can't tolerate constant digs about your decision. Call it like you see it and tell your significant other it's rude if he or she relentlessly makes jokes or gives you an underhanded hard time.

On a practical level, regardless of your gender, you need only a few basic skills and a little common kitchen equipment to manage a very healthy diet. For those who need help with kitchen skills, the following section is for you.

Basic kitchen equipment—You don't need much

Before you can really get a good start in the kitchen, you need some basic equipment. One of the most useful and versatile pieces of kitchen equipment is a blender. All you need to operate one is a good strong button-pushing finger and electricity. It's very simple.

A good chef's knife is also important as are a good paring knife and a vegetable peeler. You should be able get all these, including the blender, for less than $75.

My personal favorite for an economical yet highly reliable blender that works great is the Ninja line. These often come with a mini-food processor, which is nice to have because it does things the blender can't do so well.

You need some pans. A good-sized skillet with a lid, a saucepan or two, a stock pot, a baking dish, and a steamer (or a steamer basket for your larger saucepan or stock pot) are the basics. These should be stainless steel, glass, or enamel—no Teflon or other non-stick coatings, please. These coatings leach chemicals into your food that can be quite hazardous. This stuff is already banned in some countries.

Other useful tools include a cutting board, a grater, a coffee grinder (not just for coffee), and a juice machine. The juice machine is a more expensive purchase. I like the Jack LaLanne model well enough for those who need to economize and don't have serious health conditions. I prefer the Champion or the Green Star for those who can't afford not to be more serious about their equipment. These two gear-driven machines produce a much higher quality juice, and they last for years and years.

Now that you have some equipment to work with, what can you do with it? As we said, there are six categories of food preparation that can help you achieve awesome health. Knowing how to work with these six food preparation categories is the best way to answer that nagging "what can I eat?" question and get rid of the dietary stress in your life.

If they aren't already there, there will soon be food prep videos on my website illustrating these six methods of food preparation. Four of these methods use raw foods, two involve cooking, one can go either way. Already, you can see how this arrangement supports your efforts to incorporate more raw foods and cross over to the winning side of the 50-yard food line.

How do you stock your pantry and fridge?

Every diet has its staples. I recommend keeping plenty of the following on hand to be sure you always have options. Some of these are categories, not specific ingredients, because you need to suit your own tastes. In addition to these, there will be little extras that you like. Having plenty of these foods on hand will allow you to make everything described in the rest of this chapter.

Lettuces	Tomatoes	Extra virgin coconut oil
Kale/Greens	Avocados	Extra virgin olive oil
Fresh broccoli	Frozen fruits	Coconut manna
Fresh beets	Fresh fruits	Grape seed oil
Organic apples	Carrots	Red / yellow bell peppers
Bananas	Potatoes	Sweet potatoes
Onions	Oatmeal	Cucumbers
Garlic	Brown rice	Frozen veggies you like
Nuts/seeds you like	Whole grain tortillas	Fresh fruits you like
Oatmeal	Quinoa or couscous	Whole grain pasta
Almond butter	Raw honey	Sucanat or maple syrup
Basic spices you like	Fresh parsley	Almond or coconut milk
Butternut or acorn	squashes	Real Salt/Celtic grey sea salt
Balsamic and apple cider vinegars		

Probably the only thing on the list you've never heard of is sucanat, and it's not essential. It's what you get when you juice a sugar cane plant and let the juice dry into granules. All the original nutrients are still there, which accounts for its rich brown color. Sucanat is available in bulk in many health food stores. You can also order it online.

Everything on this list can be found at Kroger and many other major grocery stores, except for the sucanat, Celtic or Real Salt, and Coconut Manna. Those items can be found online or at most health food stores.

If you don't already know where your local health food store is, you probably need to find it. Although not everything at a health food store is healthful, it's a very good place to get things you need. Most health food stores are willing to special order things for you when they don't normally carry them. If you don't see what you need, don't hesitate to ask.

Six pillars of AWESOME nutrition

The six pillars of AWESOME Nutrition are: salads, fresh fruits and smoothies, soups, juices, healthy starches, and steamed vegetables. Better than a menu plan you must adhere to, better than a recipe book you never seem to have all the right ingredients for, these broad categories help you make the most of what's on hand and figure out what's to eat. Let's take them one at a time.

1. Salads

A salad is not just a plate full of lettuce and assorted oddments drowning in dressing. It is an appealing combination of fresh vegetables and occasionally fruits, nuts, seeds, dried fruits or veggies, etc.

Be aware that the downfall of most salads is the dressing. Most commercial dressings are extremely unhealthy. The base for any dressing is generally an oil, and it's nearly always a bad one. Soybean oil and partially hydrogenated oils are what you find on most labels.

If you can't make your own dressing, try Bragg's Healthy dressings. You can find these in the health food section at many national grocery store chains as well as at most health food stores. These dressings use a higher quality olive oil as a base and are better for you.

Everybody's had a typical salad before, but there are ways to make it better and there are also ways to break free of the traditional salad bar and do something entirely different. Let's start with some basic rules for creating a salad you can really make a meal of.

• The AWESOME green salad

1.   No iceberg lettuce—it's practically an anti-nutrient. The foundation of a good green salad is about two cups of chopped, high-quality leafy greens such as romaine lettuce, spring mix, arugula, spinach, and kale.

2.   Vary the taste by choosing different combinations of other nutrient-dense veggies to complement your greens. The choices are nearly endless as nearly any veggie can be eaten raw. Consider tomatoes, celery, cucumbers, carrots, and beets; but also raw green beans, asparagus tips, corn, snap peas, snow peas, and red bell peppers. Focusing on just a few of these for each salad will allow you to change things up and enjoy different flavors.

3.   Choose a healthy fat source for each salad. Some vitamins and minerals are fat-soluble. That means you can't use them unless there is fat available to help you absorb them. Avocados, sunflower seeds, crushed almonds, pecans, walnuts, hazelnuts, and hemp seeds are good choices.

4.   Try something different instead of bottled dressings. Flax oil is very good for you, providing lots of essential fatty acids that are hard to find elsewhere in your diet. A big spoonful on a salad will combine with the other flavors and function as dressing, especially if you have some fresh fruit on your salad. Fresh berries, kiwi, apple, or pear are great on salads. A splash of vinegar

can add that final kick of flavor you need. Try balsamic, apple cider, ume plum, or champagne vinegar when you need a change.

Personally, I don't think I could eat a large green salad every day—it just wouldn't appeal to me. Fortunately, there are lots of other ways to enjoy fresh produce. Many different combinations of veggies and seasonings can provide the variety you need, and there is a method to combining. Experiment within this framework to come up with your own unique dishes. You'll never be bored again!

- Fresh Food Combos
  1. Pick out a couple or three veggies you think would taste good together and wash, peel, chop or grate—whatever is appropriate.
  2. Select something to give the dish a foundational flavor. Vinegars, high quality oils, lemon juice, and lime juice are good for this purpose.
  3. Add some herbs to enhance the flavor. Basil, oregano, cumin, garlic, onion, fresh parsley, fresh cilantro, and Celtic sea salt are all good choices.

- Sample Recipes
  1. Tomato-Cucumber Salad
     Chopped tomatoes and cucumbers with a little olive oil, a dash of lemon juice, a bit of garlic, onion, and basil make a nice dish.
  2. Raw Green Beans Italiano
     Raw green beans with a few cherry tomatoes, some kalamata olive bits, diced onion, and a splash of balsamic vinegar and olive oil is a very tasty side. Very young green beans picked when they're no bigger around than a pencil are best for raw eating.

- Got left-overs?
  Both of the recipe ideas above are great on green salads.

Lots of veggies can be eaten raw, and an endless combination of seasonings make them taste terrific. Most raw veggie recipes like these can be made in large batches in just a few minutes, and they'll keep in the fridge for several days. Make one dish each day, and you'll always have several options to choose from and meals will be a snap. This is faster than hamburger helper!

- Make Your Own Salad Bar—It's Easy!

Without exception, the best salad tip I've ever seen comes from Hallelujah Acres (www.hacres.com). They suggest the salad box—a salad bar right in your own refrigerator. I use it myself, and it is by far the most useful tool I've found in healthy eating.

If you measure one of the shelves in your fridge, you can find two plastic containers at your local discount store that will fill that space. Wash them thoroughly and line one with waxed paper. Fill the other with short 8 or 16 ounce Mason jars. (Bigger jars for a bigger fridge and a bigger family.)

In the waxed-paper bin, put your washed and dried lettuces and greens. A salad spinner is a great asset when you need to dry lettuce. Fill the Mason jars with a variety of prepared salad ingredients you like. These can be single items like chopped tomatoes, or recipes like the raw green bean dish on the previous page. Our box often contains fresh raw corn, chopped tomatoes, sliced cucumbers, shredded carrots, marinated beets, diced green onions, chopped avocados with lime juice, and asparagus tips.

When it's meal time, you can whip these boxes out and have an instant meal in minutes. There are lots of ways to use these ingredients, especially if you also keep a supply of whole grain tortillas on top of the lettuce box. You can use the salad box ingredients to make a salad, or to augment a sandwich, or just fix up a plate lunch of raw veggie dishes. You can use the tortillas to make a fresh veggie pizza (cooks in less than 10 minutes) or a veggie burrito (heating up some beans is a nice touch).

This is a super handy way to make eating raw veggies easy. Even clean-up is simple—those mason jars fit nicely in the dishwasher! Jars are rinsed out and refilled as needed so the job doesn't get too big. When we start on empty, we each take three or four jars and soon have them filled up and ready to go. Division of labor and batch preparation are two of the keys to making this healthy lifestyle work for you.

2. Smoothies and fresh fruits

What could be easier than a smoothie? Only a piece of fresh fruit the way nature intended it. Easy to fix, easy to eat, and so portable! You can use fresh fruits or smoothies as a healthy snack, a quick nutritious breakfast, or even a whole meal in a cup.

If you're having a hard time getting started on diet reform, this is a great place to begin. Adding one piece of fresh fruit each morning is a start. As you make small additions to your diet, they begin to crowd out less healthy items. Before you know it, you're eating a lot better—and feeling better, too.

There aren't many rules where fresh fruits and smoothies are concerned, but here are a few basic principles to get you started.

- Using fresh fruit
  1. Some people believe they "can't eat fruit." Usually, this is a sign of a seriously compromised digestive system or a bad food-combination

situation. Fruits don't digest well in the presence of cooked foods. If you have trouble with fresh fruits, try eating them first thing in the morning on an empty stomach. Don't eat anything else for an hour— give the fruit time to move through your stomach before putting anything else in. Melons are loners. If you have trouble with melons, eat them alone, or leave them off the menu.

2. Fruits are nutritious, but you can overdo them. Too much, even of a good thing, isn't a good thing. Because they are high in natural sugar content, it's best to be conservative; especially if you have blood sugar problems already. Spread out your fruit intake over the morning so all the sugar doesn't hit your system all at once.

- Making the perfect smoothie

1. Choose your base. It takes some liquid to make a blender turn. Some popular choices include almond milk—which you can make at home or buy at the store, coconut milk, coconut water, apple juice, and orange or grapefruit juice. It usually doesn't take a lot of liquid to make a single serving. It depends a lot on how thick you want your shake to be.

2. Choose your thickness. You can make anything from a juice-like beverage to a soft-serve ice cream right in your blender. It's all about what ingredients you use. If you want it very thick, like ice cream, use frozen fruit. If you want it thinner, use non-frozen. A creamier consistency comes from using half an avocado.

3. Choose your ingredients. What taste do you want? Using all fruits is a fruity taste, of course. If you crave some chocolate, try grinding some raw cacao nibs in the coffee grinder and adding those or use a spoonful of carob powder. Stevia can give an extra sweet boost, and the nutrition content of almost any smoothie can be enhanced by adding alfalfa sprouts, clover sprouts, wheat or barley grass powder, or spinach. Sounds like it might taste bad, but it doesn't. The taste of the fruit is strong enough to overcome the veggies. Even your kids will drink it—if you don't tell them!

4. Blend and enjoy. Drink it with a straw or eat it from a bowl with a spoon. It's always delicious and refreshing. If you use avocado and make it thick, it's also very filling, and a smoothie of 16 ounces or so with some green ingredients definitely qualifies as a meal.

5. Adding flax oil, hemp seeds, or fresh coconut is a good way to get healthy fats into your diet. As with salads, some nutrients are dependent on the presence of fats, so it's always good to have a source of fat in your smoothie. A tablespoon of flax oil or hemp seed is plenty.

Coconut is hard to measure, but ¼ cup of fresh coconut pieces or two tablespoons of dried grated coconut is enough. Avoid sulfites.

- Sample recipes to get you started: (If you don't have these ingredients, substitute something else! You can't do it wrong!)

    1. Banana blueberry bliss—
    1 banana
    1 C frozen blueberries
    ½ C coconut water or milk
    2 medjool dates OR 1 t raw honey OR 4 drops stevia

    2. Grapefruit supreme
    1 grapefruit. Cut the pieces into the blender and squeeze in the juice
    ½ C frozen raspberries
    1 C fresh baby spinach
    2 medjool dates OR 1 t raw honey OR 4 drops stevia
    ½ avocado
    1 fresh pear

There are infinitely many combinations. If you keep an ample supply of fresh and frozen fruits on hand, you can always make a smoothie. There is almost no combination that won't work. Try it with whatever you have. You really don't need a recipe!

One word of caution: many frozen fruit suppliers sugar-coat their products. Look for packages that have no added sugar and certainly no artificial sweeteners.

- Got left-overs?

Most groceries and discount stores sell popsicle makers. If you make a little more smoothie than will fit in your glass, pour it into a popsicle maker and stick it in the freezer. It's a very healthy treat for your kids, or even for yourself. I'll never tell!

3. Soups

For many of us, soups are the ultimate comfort: warm and delicious and easy to eat. Surprise, surprise, this is the category that can be raw or cooked! Though few people have ever tried them, there are a variety of tasty raw soups that can increase your nutrient and enzyme intake and expand your menu options. We'll talk about both.

Making soup from scratch may seem a little intimidating, but it's not so hard with a few guidelines.

- How to make a good, homemade soup
  1. The foundation of every good soup is the stock. While making homemade soup stock is certainly a good thing to do, there are some easier, faster options as well. There are several brands of prepared soup stock that are organic, vegetarian, and quite good. Choosing a low sodium variety is also best. Figure on using 1—3 cups more liquid than solid ingredients depending on how thick you want your soup.
  2. If you want a primary ingredient soup or a variety soup, that will affect the rest of the recipe. A primary ingredient soup features a single primary flavor enhanced by other lesser flavors. Examples include potato soup, carrot soup, or butternut squash soup. The key to primary ingredient soups is to keep it very simple. If you put in everything you can think of every time you make a soup, all your soups will taste like variety soups. They'll all taste the same. Let the flavor of your star vegetable shine through and enjoy it. Let it be itself. Most veggies can hold their own with a minimum of accompaniment—a little celery and some onion are usually just about all you need.

     Variety soups don't have a signature flavor. Their essence is their wide variety of ingredients. Examples include classic vegetable soup, minestrone, and gazpacho. This is where you can throw everything you've got into the pot. If you like it, that's all that counts.
  3. Add your vegetables in cook time order. If something needs to be pre-cooked, you need to do that first. Apart from that, some ingredients, such as lima beans, need to cook longer than others, such as fresh white potatoes. Add those long-cooking ingredients early. Fresh, delicate ingredients such as spinach should be added at the last minute lest they disintegrate.
  4. For the sake of maximizing nutrition, consider whether there are ingredients in this soup that could be added raw after the soup is already done cooking. Tomatoes, grated carrot, and spinach can often be handled this way.
  5. Choose spices carefully, and don't overdo it. If you use more than three or four spices, you're probably cluttering your flavor. Seasoning food is like watercolor painting. If you mix any two or three colors you usually get something fairly attractive. If you mix more than that it always just turns brown. Start with basic familiar flavors like basil, oregano, parsley, and garlic. Expand your repertoire gradually, taking occasional suggestions from cookbooks you like.

6. Don't overcook. Test vegetables every few minutes for doneness. Few soups really need more than 25 or 30 minutes of cook time.

- Raw soups

The instructions for cooked soups largely also apply to raw soups —except for the bit about cooking. There are a few raw food prep books and websites offering recipes for raw soups and other foods, and I would recommend working from a recipe the first few times you try a raw soup. Raw soups are usually either very good or very bad. There doesn't seem to be much middle ground. Most raw soups are prepared in a blender and served at room temperature or just slightly warmed on the stove. If you choose to warm it, keep the burner very low and don't stop stirring. You wouldn't want to go to the trouble of making and eating a raw soup when it wasn't actually raw!

- Sample recipes

    1. Butternut squash soup (cooked)
        1 large butternut squash, peeled, seeded, and cubed
        1 large carrot
        1 small or ½ large sweet yellow onion
        2 stalks of celery
        1 carton of low-sodium vegetable broth
        Extra water as needed
        Cook all the ingredients. Add as much water as you need to thin it as desired. Blend and serve. A hand-blender works well for this soup.

    2. Gazpacho (It's raw!)

        Blend these ingredients, serve, and enjoy!

        5 ripe tomatoes, peeled and chopped
        ½ purple onion, diced
        1 stalk celery
        2 T fresh parsley
        1 T fresh cilantro
        1 T fresh chives
        ½ red bell pepper, seeded and chopped
        ½ C chopped cucumber
        small clove garlic
        2 T red wine vinegar
        ½ small lemon (juice from)
        1 t honey
        3 drops of Tabasco sauce (optional)
        ½ t soy sauce or Bragg's Liquid Aminos

2 T extra-virgin olive oil
Salt and pepper as needed

- Got left-overs?

Great! Soups store well in Mason jars and keep for several days. You can also freeze them for several months in single servings, share them with a friend, take them to work for lunch tomorrow in your thermos, or just have another bowl.

One note about soups. It's well-known that people who eat soup more often lose weight more efficiently than those who don't. Maybe it's because there is good nutrition in soup. Maybe it's because the extra water content helps you feel full faster. Maybe it's all that and more. In any case, soup is an easy meal to fix for yourself or for a crowd, and it goes so well with a salad!

4. Juices

Juice can be the cornerstone of your nutritional arsenal. You can live on juice—literally. A diet of fresh juices, salads, smoothies and fresh fruits, and an occasional raw soup would really be excellent. In fact, you should consider these four the cornerstones of a really solid raw plant-based diet. Everything else is the icing on the cake.

- What do you need to know about juicing? Not much.

    1. There are two kinds of juice machines. The graters and the grinders. Graters look like graters—they have a basket-like apparatus at the top that spins the juice out. Grinders have one or two gears that crush the vegetables to release the juice. Grinders are more expensive, but produce higher quality and quantity of juice. Graters cause a lot of oxidation which means nutrient loss. They also don't extract as much juice from your veggies, so they often cost more in the long run.

    2. Organic carrots are an absolute necessity for juicing. There is no comparison in taste. I find the taste of non-organic carrot juice so offensive I literally can't get it down. This is not true of all veggies, just carrots.

    3. Carrots are usually the base for vegetable juice combinations. You can try it with tomatoes, but they tend to clog your juice machine. It's easier to blend a tomato and strain the juice than to run a tomato through your juice machine.

    4. Dark leafy lettuces and greens make very healthy juice, but it's very potent and you don't need much of it.

5. Beet juice is also a very potent juice. Two ounces of beet juice in a day is enough for most people. Don't be alarmed, beet juice will turn urine pink, among other things. There is no harm in this.

6. Juice will keep in the fridge overnight, but the taste deteriorates quickly and so does the nutrient content.

7. Some people find that their skin takes on a slight orange cast after they have juiced for a little while. If everyone were eating as they should, we'd all be orange. You're not the abnormal one. Don't let anyone get away with telling you there's something wrong with being a little orange. Be orange and be proud. It's a good healthy color.

8. It takes about 10 medium carrots to make an 8 oz glass of juice. One medium apple will give you about 4 ounces.

9. Never walk away from your juice machine without cleaning it! You'll be sorry later.

10. Using a fine strainer for your juice will make it smooth and more appealing.

- Good juice combinations:

10 organic carrots	Makes 12—14 oz.
1 small apple	
1 stalk of celery	
½ red bell pepper	
8 organic carrots	Makes about 12 oz.
1 small apple	
1 handful of fresh parsley or cilantro	
1 sliver of fresh ginger	
1 large apple	Makes about 6 oz.
½ medium-large beet	
1 sliver of fresh ginger	
2 T lemon juice	

- Got leftovers?

Just drink it. It doesn't keep well. If you can't drink it all, you can also use it as a base for certain raw soups or you can share it with someone you love.

5. Healthy starches

Healthy starches include root vegetables like white potatoes and sweet potatoes, hard squashes, and whole grains. Although there are important nutrients in these foods, the nutrient-to-calorie ratio isn't as strong as it is in green veggies, fresh fruits, or juices. Starches are more calorie dense than most other healthy foods, and they are usually cooked, so limiting these is necessary if optimal health is your goal.

There are other vegetables that are less starchy and more nutrient dense than the potatoes and squashes. These include beets, carrots, and parsnips, and they all go very well in combination recipes with the heavier starches, which increases the nutritional value of your meal.

If you struggle with hunger issues while trying to eat a healthy diet, you'll find some relief in the starch category. These foods will make you feel full, and the extra calorie density slows things down so you aren't hungry again quite so soon.

There are two subcategories here, grains and veggies. Of the two, starchy veggies have a little more to offer in the way of nutrition. Here's a short list of possible ways to enjoy some starchy vegetables.

Baked sweet potatoes

Baked white potatoes

Baked acorn, butternut, or spaghetti squashes

Creamy soups made from those squashes

Stir-fried spaghetti squash "noodles"

Mashed potatoes

Mashed sweet potatoes

Oven-roasted seasoned potatoes

Oven-roasted seasoned sweet potatoes

Oven-roasted combination of beets, parsnips, carrots, & potatoes

These sound pretty good. The problem area is what to put on those starchy veggies. When most of us envision our favorite starchy vegetables, there are usually accompanying visions of butter, sour cream, and brown sugar involved as well. Without those, the thrill is gone. Are there any worthy substitutes?

Yes and no. Nobody is perfect, but if you are going to cheat, do it with butter not margarine. Margarine, no matter what they say, contains altered fats that will do you wrong one way and another—far more wrong than butter ever will.

If you just have to have some butter, please use organic. The pesticides, antibiotics, and hormones used in non-organic dairy and beef production are concentrated in the meat and dairy products. Meat is the single richest source for these contaminants in the American diet. If you really want to reduce your chemical load, cut the meat and dairy, not the fruits and veggies.

- How do you prepare healthy starchy vegetables?

  1. Choose your vegetable(s). One interesting thing about starchy vegetables is that they all go well together. Almost no combination will disappoint you. Choose one, two, or several based on how much time you want to spend in the kitchen and what you have on hand.

  2. Bake or roast, don't fry. There is nothing you can do with a starchy vegetable in a frying pan that you can't do better in the oven. Get high quality grape seed oil, which is about the only economical choice that can tolerate high heat without becoming harmful, and use it sparingly to create the "fried feel" you are used to without all the bad oil.

  3. Add some seasonings. The best way to learn to season food properly is to skim through some recipe books to see what types of seasonings usually go with specific types of foods. Here's a short list to get you started:

     • Basil, oregano, fennel, garlic, and onion are generally associated with Italian style cooking. They go well with pasta, rice, and tomato-based soups, but also with white potatoes.

     • Chili powder, cayenne, cumin, and onion are usually associated with Mexican-style cooking. They go well with white potatoes, beans, soups, and burritos, but also on fresh corn (don't cook it, it's delicious raw).

     • Rosemary, thyme, bay leaf, and onion complement soups and pot pies where a slightly sweeter flavor is desired.

  4. Baking time depends on how hot your oven is, and how small the pieces of vegetable are cut. Smaller veggies and hotter ovens mean shorter baking times. Keep this in mind when you need to speed things up, but don't bake your uncovered veggies at more than 375 degrees—you'll brown them too much, too fast.

  5. To cover or not to cover, that is the question, and it's primarily a question of texture. If you want a crisper or firmer texture with a little browning, uncovered is essential. If you want it really soft and moist, covered is the only way to go.

  6. Aluminum foil may make cleanup a snap, but it's not good for you in the long run. Aluminum leaches out of the foil and into your food. Aluminum is a potent neurotoxin which can seriously affect the health of your brain and nervous system. Vegetables, even whole potatoes, should be baked in a covered glass dish. Leave the foil out of the equation.

7. In a pinch, foil covering a dish is a lesser evil than foil in direct contact with your food. Condensation will still cause aluminum-laden water to drip into your food, so it's not a great solution. It's better if you use a piece of waxed paper between the foil and the food to block some of the condensation. Make sure the waxed paper is fully covered by the foil, however, because it could create smoke or even a fire hazard if the waxed paper is too close to the heating element.

8. Skin off or skin on, that is the other question. The answer depends on the vegetable and your preferences. If you are cooking organic veggies, skin on is always an option. You don't eat the skin of a hard squash, organic or not, but many enjoy the skins of white and sweet potatoes and there is good nutrition there—if you plan to eat the skin, get an organic tater. Large, thick-skinned squashes are very hard to peel. It's easier to cook them with the skin still on and scoop out the vegetable with a spoon afterwards. Cutting a hard squash in half will help it to cook far more quickly.

- Simple sample recipes

    1. Baked sweet potato
        1 large sweet potato
        2 T coconut manna
        2 t organic maple syrup or raw honey
        ½ t coriander

        Bake the potato in a covered dish at 375 degrees for 45 minutes. Mix the other ingredients together. When the sweet potato is done, split it open and top it with the spread

    2. Roasted root vegetables
        2 large russet potatoes
        2 long carrots
        1 large beet
        1 parsnip
        ½ medium sweet onion
        1 large clove garlic
        4 T grape seed oil
        2 t basil
        1 t oregano
        1 small handful fresh parsley

        Peel and chop the veggies. Add them to a 9x13 glass pan. Drizzle the oil over the vegetables. Sprinkle on the spices. Stir well. Bake uncovered at 350 degrees for 45–60 minutes.

- A word about breads and whole grains

Grains are the other half of the starch category. By now, we don't even need to mention that we're only using whole grains, right? But you need to become proficient at reading labels. Things labeled "natural" seldom are as that word has no official meaning other than "found somewhere in universe."

While we're on the subject of grains, let's clear up a major misconception. Many people don't understand that white bread is still made from wheat flour. Wheat flour can be refined (also called white) or whole grain (often called wheat). Both flours started out as identical wheat plants side by side in the same field. There is no such thing as a "white plant" used to make white flour. White flour is wheat flour with the nutrients removed. That's why it's white now; the nutrients are gone, and only the starch is left.

Whole wheat bread isn't always what you think either. It is perfectly legal, though entirely unethical, to fool the public with terms like wheat and whole wheat when, in fact, there is much refined flour in the product. If something doesn't specifically say 100% whole grain wheat, it isn't.

Bread is an important issue. Most commonly available brands are really harmful to your health. Bromine, regardless of what form it's in, is part of the same chemical family as iodine. Fluorine (fluoride) is part of the family also.

When you consume fluorine or bromine, they displace iodine from its vital role in your body, and bromine, in one form or another, is almost always in commercially produced bread. Thyroid malfunction is rampant in America. Your thyroid function is totally dependent on your iodine supply.

If thyroid dysfunction isn't incriminating enough, the EPA has also listed potassium bromide as a carcinogen, yet it's still added to most of the bread commercially produced in this country. Check the loaf in your kitchen.

Making your own bread from freshly ground or sprouted grains is ideal, but not realistic for most people. A very good substitute is Ezekiel Bread. Ask your grocery store if they have it or are willing to get it. Many Kroger stores and health food stores now carry this regularly. There are several varieties and all are very good. They are generally in the health food frozen food section of the store, but you keep them in the fridge once you get them home.

Ezekiel bread is a cut above most any other, not only because it tastes good and is made from whole organic grains and seeds with no chemicals, but also because the grains and seeds are sprouted, making the nutrients more bioavailable for you. For those who still get excited by the prospect of a more "complete" protein, this bread contains 18 amino acids.

How do you cook with whole grains? There are lots of ways to use whole grains in a healthy diet. Brown rice and whole grain pasta are familiar to most of us and easy to use. Instructions are right on the package, and everybody knows what to put with these—stir-fried veggies for the rice and a tomato-based sauce or some sautéed veggies for the pasta.

If you have tried whole grain pasta and brown rice in the past and had bad luck, try using a slightly shorter cooking time for non-wheat pastas and slightly less water with rice than what is called for on the package.

Another very important note about cooking brown rice: to prevent stickiness, you need to do three things. First, add a tablespoon of grape seed oil to your pan and sauté the rice in that for about one minute before adding the water. Second, once you add the water, you never stir the rice. Third, when rice is done cooking, take it off the burner but leave the lid on for ten more minutes. These three tips should make you a pro when it comes to cooking good brown rice.

We're also familiar with good old-fashioned oatmeal, and we've already talked about breads. Other possibilities are less well-known. Most any fresh whole grain can be ground up, often in your coffee grinder, and cooked like oatmeal to make a cereal. This is very handy information for those who are gluten or corn intolerant. Millet can be substituted anywhere corn meal or grits are called for to make things like cream of millet cereal or millet "corn" bread for those who can't eat wheat or corn.

A relative newcomer to the American dietary scene, quinoa is already gathering many fans. This grain is actually a seed, and it's a great option for the gluten intolerant. It's also a great option when you want rice but don't have time. Quinoa can be used in any way you might use rice, but it is fully cooked and ready to serve in less than 15 minutes. The nutritional profile of quinoa is superior to all the grains mentioned here. It has a nice variety of vitamins and minerals, a lower carbohydrate count than most grains, plenty of fiber, and all the essential amino acids—which is nice, but isn't necessary. Use 2 cups of liquid for every cup of dry quinoa, boil it for 12—15 minutes and enjoy.

Polenta is yet another useful concoction. It can be substituted for pasta, in a few recipes, or it can stand alone. It's basically like a very thick bowl of corn grits—so thick you can cut it with a knife. You can store it in the fridge rolled in waxed paper sausage style, and slice off what you need. You can buy it pre-made or make it yourself.

If you sauté polenta in a dab of coconut or grape seed oil, it can be topped with almost anything from tomato sauce to ratatouille. It can even be substituted for lasagna noodles to make a delicious, though not multilayered, vegetable lasagna.

Couscous is another whole grain option, and this one is super fast and easy. Think of couscous as noodles crushed into tiny bits, and use it anywhere you would use noodles or as a really fast substitute for brown rice. To prepare it, measure out the couscous into a glass or stainless steel bowl and add boiling water or broth. Cover it for five to ten minutes and it's ready. It generally takes 2-3 times as much water as couscous. Check the directions when you buy it. Not all couscous is whole wheat, some is refined, so watch out for that.

Corn bread or millet bread can also be used as a base for all sorts of creations. Corn bread tends to work well with recipes featuring beans of all kinds, such as "Mexican pizza," but it can also be used as a base for delicious vegetable pies.

Although there certainly are plenty of fancy ways to use whole grains, most of the time simple wins out just because we don't have a lot of time to spend in the kitchen. When you think about what to eat at any given meal, it's probably best to start with what's easy. Oatmeal, whole grain corn grits, basic hot cereals, pre-made polenta, couscous, brown rice, and pasta are all really simple additions to a healthy meal that will meet your calorie needs without robbing you of nutrients. Many of these can be made ahead of time or in large batches and kept for several days to make meals even easier and faster.

There are so many differences between whole grain products it's impossible to list specific instructions that would be accurate across the board, but there are a few principles to be aware of.

1. Most whole grain products will be cooked in liquid, but it doesn't have to be water. The nutrient count for rice, quinoa, pasta, corn grits, millet, and couscous goes up considerably if you cook these in broth or soup stock, and the taste improves exponentially. The whole idea behind maximizing nutrition is to add nutritional value everywhere you can to keep the balance between nutrients and calories clearly skewed in favor of nutrients.

2. Textures in whole grain cooking are generally a function of the water-to-dry-ingredient ratio. If your grain is too sticky, try less water or try leaving the lid on for a while after cooking. If your grain is too hard, you need a bit more water, or you need to use a tight-fitting lid.

3. With pasta, it's all about time. Longer cooking time means softer pasta. If you detect a residue you don't like, shorten the cooking time a little or rinse the pasta after it's cooked to get rid of excess starch.

4. If you want an unusually thick product, like polenta, you still need to start with the right amount of water, but you'll need to cook it longer—until all the excess water evaporates and you achieve the desired consistency.

5. Many grain products continue to soak up water and expand after cooking is over. If you've finished cooking and you think it's still too thin, let it sit and cool a while and you may be surprised how thick it gets. Conversely, if you get it just like you want it while it's cooking, you may not be happy with it later. Just remember, you can always thin it down if necessary.

- Sample Recipes
  1. Homemade Polenta
     2 C corn grits (or ground millet)
     6 C water or broth
     1 t Celtic gray sea salt

     Bring water and salt to a boil. Slowly add corn grits, whisking constantly with a wire whisk for about one minute to prevent lumps. Cover with a tight-fitting lid, and simmer on low heat for about 30 minutes.

     When it's done, spread it in a greased 9x13 pan and bake it for 10 minutes at 350 degrees to use it as a crust for a pot pie or a Mexican pizza. Polenta is wonderful in the bottom of a bowl of your favorite hot soup. Left-over polenta, lightly sautéed, makes an interesting addition to your breakfast plate. You can also serve it just as it is.

     If you make extra, you can let it cool, spoon it onto a large sheet of waxed paper, roll it into a thick log shape, wrap it in plastic wrap and store it in the fridge for up to 4 days. As you need it, you can slice it and sauté it lightly for plain eating or as a crust for other things.

  2. AWESOME Old-Fashioned Oatmeal, made easy
     1/3 C organic quick-cooking rolled oats
     1 C water
     2 t sucanat*
     dash of cinnamon
     tiny pinch of sea salt
     Put the dry ingredients in a sturdy, heat-resistant bowl. Boil the water. Pour the water over the dry ingredients. Let it sit for 5 minutes. Add raisins, sunflower seeds, crushed almonds, or other things you like.

     You can use this recipe to prepare your own "instant" oatmeal packets. Just put all the dry ingredients in a snack-sized, air-tight plastic bag. Make several packets in just a few minutes. These keep for weeks.

* Sucanat is what you get when you juice a sugar cane plant and dry the juice. It still has all the nutrients of the original plant. You can buy this product at most health food stores, often in bulk. If you can't find it, use organic maple syrup instead—after you cook the oatmeal, of course!

- Got Left-overs?

Many, though not all, grain and pasta products will keep for several days in the fridge and can be used later as small portions or additions to other recipes. For example, a little leftover brown rice or quinoa makes a nice addition to a bean burrito or a green salad. You might want to add a little rice or pasta to a hearty vegetable soup. Store left-over polenta in the fridge and use it as described above.

6. Steamed and sautéed vegetables

This final category of foods is probably the area in which skill makes the biggest difference in how much you enjoy your food—and how well you manage to stick to this dietary lifestyle. It seems that most people really enjoy their meat, and then tolerate the obligatory side dish of vegetables. The primary reason for this, I believe, is the gross lack of knowledge on how to prepare vegetables properly. When you do them right, vegetables are absolutely beautiful and delicious. When you do them wrong, they can really be disgusting.

In preparation for cooking vegetables you need two things. First, make sure you have a really large skillet with a tight-fitting lid. Second, make sure you have either a vegetable steamer or a deep pan with a steamer basket you can put inside it, with a tight-fitting lid. These steamer baskets are expandable to fit most pans, and they are available at a reasonable cost at most stores where cooking supplies are sold.

In this section, you'll learn methods that work to make any vegetable look and taste fantastic and still retain substantial nutritional value. The best part is, it's so easy!

- How do you prepare steamed or sautéed vegetables?

  1. Take your microwave oven to the nearest Goodwill Store. There is no better way to utterly ruin the taste of any vegetable than to nuke it. No nukes!

  2. The first rule for making vegetables taste great is to buy fresh, high quality vegetables. Some frozen veggies are okay, but fresh is always best. Some veggies just have to start fresh if they are to turn out right. These include broccoli, asparagus, spinach, and all other leafy greens, and brussels sprouts. If you're saying "No way I'm eating those..."

I'm not surprised. You've probably never had them made from fresh before. That's why I'm telling you, buy these fresh or not at all!

3. Peppers, onions, green beans, lima beans, and cauliflower are tolerable frozen. They still are better fresh, but to save time, it's okay to buy them frozen. Just make sure there is nothing in the package except the vegetables. Special sauces tend to be full of unhealthy ingredients.

4. Never cook a frozen veggie in the bag it came in—even if the bag says to do it. It won't taste very good unless it's slathered in special sauce which is absolutely sure to be really bad for you.

5. Potatoes and dried beans are prepared by boiling; other veggies should never be boiled. Boiling leaches vitamins and minerals out of the veggies and into the water, which you'll likely throw away.

6. Sauté broccoli, cauliflower, green beans, asparagus, peppers, and summer squashes. When you sauté, start by putting a little oil such as coconut or grape seed in the skillet first to keep food from sticking. Use a little broth or water to keep the food from burning to the pan and to create steam. Add more as needed, but don't float your food —that's boiling. When you put the lid on your sauté pan, you are steam sautéing your veggies. That's fine, just be aware of what effect you're having on the texture. Steam sautéing produces a more tender texture than plain sautéing.

7. Carrots and parsnips are best prepared by steaming.

8. Beets are best prepared in a covered dish in the oven or by steaming.

9. Peas can be prepared by dropping them in boiling water for one minute, then draining them. They can also be steamed or sautéed.

10. You should prepare the pan first and add the veggies when the pan is hot for sautéing, or when the water is boiling for steaming.

11. Steaming doesn't require an excess of water, but it does require a tight-fitting lid to keep the water, and nutrients, in there.

12. Seasoning matters. Experiment with a variety of herbs and vinegars to achieve tastes that please you. Balsamic, champagne, apple cider, and ume plum are several vinegars you commonly find in stores that offer a wide variety of tastes. Fresh herbs such as parsley and cilantro are also readily and cheaply available, and they really boost the nutritional value of your cooking. High quality organic dried herbs and spices are available at many health food stores in bulk, which means much better quality at a much lower price.

13. Some vitamins and minerals can't be absorbed without fat. Using oils in your cooking assists your body in getting the maximum nutrition out of your food. When possible, add oils after the cooking is done to preserve the good of the oil. Use only extra virgin oils. Olive, grape seed, and coconut are good oils. Avoid the others, especially canola. If you can't live without a dab of organic butter on your broccoli, I understand.

14. Don't cook things longer than necessary. Most people overcook their food. Mush is not good. A firm, slightly crisp, yet tender consistency is how vegetables want to be presented. The time it takes to achieve it varies with the vegetable. If you turn the burner off but leave the veggies in the pan, they are still cooking. Consider the following table of times for steaming or sautéing:

Leafy greens, including spinach and kale	5 –7 minutes
Young, thin green beans	8–10 minutes
Broccoli or cauliflower	10–12 minutes
Brussels sprouts	12–15 minutes, depends on size
Asparagus	3 minutes (seriously)
Peppers, onions, celery, mushrooms	5 minutes
Tomatoes and summer squash	5—8 minutes

- Sample Recipes

    1. Steam sautéed broccoli
        1 large head of broccoli
        1 T coconut oil
        ½ C vegetable broth
        sea salt or Real Salt
        Wash the broccoli and cut off the bulky stem. Chop the broccoli into bite-sized pieces. Melt the oil in the pan. Toss the broccoli in the pan to coat it with the oil. Add the broth. Cover the pan and steam for 10 minutes. Stir occasionally and don't let it go dry. Serve immediately.

    2. AWESOME Asparagus
        1 bunch of fresh asparagus
        1 -2 T coconut oil
        sea salt or Real Salt
        Wash the asparagus and cut off the bottom 1–2 inches of stem. Melt the oil in a large skillet. Put the spears in the skillet and turn them to coat them with oil. Continue to keep them moving in the hot skillet for 3 minutes. Serve immediately.

3. Bodacious Brussels Sprouts
   15—20 sprouts
   2 T coconut oil
   2 T lemon juice
   1 t sucanat
   2 T crushed hazelnuts

   Wash and trim fresh Brussels sprouts. Steam the sprouts in a steamer pan for 10–15 minutes. Remove them promptly. Place all other ingredients in a skillet. Add sprouts and stir to coat them, about one minute. Serve immediately.

- Got left-overs?

Call me! Or, just put them in a covered dish in the fridge and eat them tomorrow. Cooked veggies will keep for about three days if you put them away promptly. When you try to reheat veggies like these, it's best to do so by the same methods used to cook them originally—in a skillet or sauce pan with very little liquid and not for very long.

- Making the 6 pillars of maximum nutrition work for you

Making this system work is as simple as ordering from a restaurant. You know the menu sections—they're the six pillars we just discussed. The selections within each section come from what you have on hand at the moment. To make an entire meal, just combine sections. Some classics are soup and salad, pasta with sautéed vegetables, rice with stir-fried vegetables, two steamed veggies and a baked potato, and so on.

If you want a soup, for example, and you have a nice butternut squash, but you don't have any tomatoes, you make some squash soup. If you want a shake, but you're out of blackberries, no problem, use strawberries instead. It's easy to make substitutions within these categories based on the ingredients you actually have. Need parsley but all you have is cilantro? Just go with that.

On the next page are some sample daily menus using this system.

There are infinitely many ways to have a healthy meal and a healthy day. Do what works for you.

Eating right on the road

Eating right when you have to work outside your home can be challenging, but it's very manageable. The best way is to bring food with you. It's easy to pack a few things when you're off to work or know you'll be out for a while. A sandwich, an apple, some carrot juice, a freezer pack, and off you go. Lots of

	Day 1	Day 2	Day 3
Breakfast	Banana blueberry bliss smoothie	Fresh grapefruit, oatmeal	Fresh fruit plate with kiwi, strawberries, blackberries, banana
Lunch	Large green salad and a bowl of raw gazpacho soup	Sliced cucumbers raw green bean salad, bean/veggie burrito	Veggie pizza on a whole grain tortilla, carrot sticks, celery with almond butter
Snack	16 oz. carrot & apple juice	16 oz. carrot, celery, red bell pepper juice	16 oz. carrot, beet, apple, ginger juice
Dinner	Polenta with sauteed broccoli, black-eyed peas, tomato/cucumber salad	Brown rice, stir-fried veggies	Large green salad, baked sweet potato, bodacious brussels sprouts

other things travel well, too. Salads, burritos, smoothies in mason jars, marinated veggies, even soups in thermoses—all travel just fine. If you've got access to a fridge at work, you're really set. Stock it for two or three days at a time to make life easier.

Build a car kit

One thing that has been very helpful for us is the car kit. It's a small plastic tub in which we keep paper plates and bowls, plastic utensils, straws, cups, paper towels, a bottle of water for dampening the paper towels as needed, a shaker of Real Salt, a shaker of pepper, and some granola bars for emergencies. This kit makes it easy to eat on the go—especially with kids.

For longer trips, you've already got your car kit, and they now make coolers that are actually small refrigerators. They plug into the lighter outlet in your car. You can carry enough cold food in there to feed a family of six for three days or more. You can pack potato salad, green bean and tomato salad, all sorts of pre-washed and pre-cut veggies and fruits, hummus, coconut milk, homemade soups in mason jars, raw almond butter, guacamole, and basically anything you would keep at home.

What I would not pack in there would be things I could easily get at grocery stores and restaurants along the way. Things like cooked green beans, cooked broccoli, baked potatoes, and salads are usually easy to find wherever you go.

A box with some of those instant oatmeal packets, some cans of organic natural soups as a back-up, maybe some quinoa or couscous, pre-washed apples wrapped in plastic, homemade granola bars, whole grain cereal, and a loaf of bread should keep you going for quite a while. Even though this fare isn't as high-quality as what you can do while you're at home, it's a huge cut above the fast food most travelers rely on.

Eating at the grocery store

Another solution to the problem of eating away from home is to head for the local grocery store. Even if they don't have a salad bar, most offer a number of ready-to-eat options that are fairly healthy. Pre-washed carrots, broccoli florets, snow peas, and cauliflower, and green beans are easy to find. There are even single serving packets of pre-made guacamole or salsa you can use to dip your veggies in. Pre-cut fresh fruits are available, too. You always find a loaf of whole grain bread and usually a tub of pre-made hummus. Grab a few items from your car kit and you've got all you need for great meal.

Restaurants

If you're out longer than expected and you're unprepared that's okay. Restaurants are no problem. The 6 pillars are keyed to work off the menu system already!

If there is a decent salad bar, you're halfway there already. Add a bowl of vegetable soup or a baked potato and you're all set. Most restaurants also have a short list of vegetables you can order a la carte. Things like mustard greens, corn, green beans, broccoli, mashed potatoes, and more. Some of these have ingredients or preparation methods that aren't perfect, but you can do all right for a meal or two.

If you can't find a suitable salad dressing while you're out, try some fresh fruit on your salad. Remember also, that most all restaurants have lemon, olive oil, and balsamic vinegar which they will bring if you ask for them. You can combine these in a little dish to make a very suitable salad dressing that won't compromise your health.

Some restaurant menus aren't so vegetable-friendly, but I learned a very important lesson about eating healthy at restaurants when I first changed my diet many years ago.

We had just made major changes in our diet when something worth celebrating happened in our lives and we wanted a night out. I made a reservation at one of the best restaurants in town and, at the same time, I asked about the menu to see if we could do all right there. The selection was not good for us, and I mentioned to the hostess when we arrived that we were new vegetarians and wondered if there was anything else. She went to fetch the chef from the kitchen and I felt embarrassed—but not for long.

As it turned out, the chef was well-educated in vegetable preparation skills he seldom got to use, and he was delighted to have us. He was so excited, he fixed an entire menu just for us and visited us after each course to discuss how he had prepared it—I had mentioned that I needed to learn more about healthy cooking. When we finished about six courses of the best food we'd ever had, we were charged the lowest price on the menu. We were shocked.

The moral of the story is that a chef knows how to cook anything you need. If you don't see what you're looking for on the menu, just ask for it. Not only do they not mind, they often enjoy the change of pace (unless you're there at rush hour). You can alter standard menu items or ask for something entirely different. It's not a problem. All restaurants have vegetables, and they can easily sauté or steam them for you. All decent restaurants have olive oil and real butter, also.

Teaching children to eat healthy

Who's teaching your kids about diet and health? We object sometimes to junk food marketing aimed at kids, but I don't believe that's the problem. It's the parents who believe it and the parents who actually buy the stuff. It's the parents who believe that's the "fun" food, and it's parents who provide that junk at picnics, kids' sports events, and other social functions. The kids don't pick the menu, the parents do.

Industry tells us, the parents, that kids only like things that are purple or blue and full of sugar. It's got to have marshmallows and prizes in the box. It's got to be in a box or a really cool carton. That's nonsense! Don't you fall for that! Kids will eat healthy food if it's provided and they are taught to eat it. That's why parents have the power to say NO. Use it! You don't need to take control of the situation, you need to realize you already have it and you've been in control all along.

We all love our kids, but we also all feel guilty. When we say no and see that sad little face, we feel bad. When we see that somebody else's kid looks really happy sucking sugar-laden yogurt out of a plastic tube and our kid doesn't have one, we feel guilty. We want our kids to have everything good. The problem is that marketing gurus are taking advantage of us and sending us bad messages. You have to educate yourself to understand that all those kids on TV who look so happy eating green and purple ketchup and cereal that looks and tastes like cookies are paid to smile. They are being used to make you think that's how you can make your kids happy. It's a bunch of lies. Your kids will be happy being healthy and they'll be happy spending time with you—that's what makes kids happy. They need love, not Sweetie Flakes.

Somehow we've come to associate being a kid and having fun with bad food, and we think the consequences won't set in till later. Bad stuff is grown-up stuff—it doesn't happen to kids. Well, unfortunately, it does. Kids as young as five are now forming plaque in their arteries. Children are being medicated for high blood pressure. The rate of childhood obesity is growing rapidly, as is the rate of childhood diabetes. Children are dying on the sports fields and in the hospitals of all the same things that kill their parents and grandparents. Don't kid yourself, childhood offers no protection from the damage bad food and other bad habits can do.

Why preach so much? Because changing the way you feed your kids isn't easy and you need solid motivation. You have to be absolutely sure it matters and it's worth it. You also need solid advice on how to do it. So here we go...

What to do with your kids

The first thing you have to do is to put a stop to the most dangerous food habits. After many years of experience with my own children and children in the foster care system, I can tell you authoritatively that the chemicals in most "kid food" kills young children's appetites. With no appetite, how will you ever persuade them to eat healthy food?

These kids often look healthy and are of normal weight even though they eat only a few bites of food at each meal. This is because junk food is very rich in calories which they convert to fat, and it's also very rich in chemicals which make them hyper and suppress their hunger. They look like they have normal energy levels because of the sugar high and the adrenal buzz.

The critical nutrient-poor foods you have to stop are:

- Candy
- Pop and flavored drink mixes
- Store-bought cakes, cookies, etc
- Mixes for muffins, pancakes, cakes, and cookies
- Hot dogs and cheap pre-packaged lunch meat
- Fast food

Every child we took in came to us from places where they had almost nothing to eat but pizza, hamburgers, French fries, pop, candy, and gum. At first, we tried to make allowances for this and transition them off it, but it didn't work at all. We found their appetite so poor they didn't even eat reasonable quantities of junk food.

What did work, every time, was to completely remove the junk food from their diets and offer only fresh fruits, fresh veggies, whole grains, and water. Invariably, they spent the first two to four days feeling listless as they detoxified. They ate so little it was frightening, but they were not sick. They played a little and slept alright. We worried and wondered if a little bit of junk food wasn't better than no food at all, but on the third or fourth day their appetites would return and suddenly they were ready to eat all those wholesome foods we had been offering. These kids were very young, 2—5.

Older kids and those whose diets aren't completely horrible are more difficult. They often hold out longer. Still, if you stick to the plan and provide no junk, they will eat good food eventually. It's hard to watch them do without, but sometimes it's necessary. As long as you put plenty of good, healthy food in front of them several times daily, you aren't starving your children.

The most difficult are the teenagers. You don't have much control over what they eat when they aren't at home. The best thing to do with them is teach, teach, teach—and respect their intelligence. Call on them to make right decisions, but don't railroad them. It's fine to refuse to provide junk food, but you can't force the good food. If you win the battle by force, you'll lose the war by default.

The process of dealing effectively with children of all ages on any issue has five major components:

- Enthusiasm. Enthusiasm is contagious. If you approach change as an adventure, they will too.

- Explanation. Knowledge motivates at any age. Share what you learn in a positive and age-appropriate way.

- Example. Practice what you preach.

- Expectations. You have to make some rules and *tell them why*.

- Encouragement. You have to be sympathetic and supportive when it's hard for them, and tell them when you're proud of them for doing it right. Make sure you're on the same team—share the struggle.

If your kids are old enough, let them read this book. If they're not, read bits of it to them or explain it to them in a way they can understand. Relate food and lifestyle choices to health in ways they can relate to. "Remember when you had that bad cold last month? If you don't want that to happen again, you need to go to bed on time and not eat all these sweets." Kids have to be taught to make these cause-and-effect connections; it doesn't come naturally.

Although it's good sometimes to have an actual lesson on the 7 Keys to AWESOME Health, or maybe seven short lessons, it's important to mention facts as you go along, in the course of conversation. If this information is to become a prominent part of your life, it has to be coming up in conversation regularly—not just when you say no to something they want or when you feel like nagging.

Playing the cart game, from part 1 of chapter 6, with your kids is one way to reinforce what you're teaching and give you something to talk about on the way home. This is not meant to be an exercise in making fun of people; it's meant to be a dose of reality and a way to learn from, rather than repeat, the mistakes of others. You can teach your children to feel compassion for others and gratitude for what you're teaching them as well. It's sad and unfortunate that everyone doesn't know more about healthy living.

Obviously, nothing you say will mean much if you aren't doing what's right yourself. If you meet with much opposition, you may need to attend to this step first. You can be living proof of the good healthy habits can do.

Remember the Tom Sawyer principle. While setting a good example, you need to sell it. Make it look good, and sound good. If you talk about how restricted you feel or how much you miss the junk food or make other negative comments, it will be very hard to convince anyone else to try it and it will also undermine your efforts on your own behalf.

Rules and rewards

No parent likes rules. Not only does it make you less popular in the beginning, it's also a lot of work! Better is the rule never made than the rule never enforced. That's the absolute truth.

Believe it or not, there are a few rules for making a good rule.

1. It must be simple and clear.
2. It must not have a lot of exceptions.
3. You must thoroughly explain your reasons for it before it goes into effect.
4. You must not break it yourself.
5. You must post it where they can see it.
6. You must be compassionate in enforcement. Catching rule breakers is not a sport, and you shouldn't relish it.

Expectations have to be realistic based on the age and ability of the child. The rule is made for the child, not the child for the rule. Expectations should be adjusted as a child matures and becomes more knowledgeable and capable. Here are some examples of rules that could work for a young child (2–7) just beginning to transition from a junky diet to a healthy diet:

1. You must eat at least one raw vegetable each day.
2. You must eat at least one fresh fruit each day.
3. When we try something new, you must take at least 2 bites.

4. We will not be having candy, cake, or cookies every day.

5. You may not whine when we say no to something.

6. When people offer you candy, you will say "no thank you."

Here are a few examples of rules for older kids (8–15):

1. You may not drink pop.

2. You may not eat candy bars.

3. You must eat either a salad or some raw vegetables every day.

4. I will not buy junky cereals, pastries, or rolls that pop out of tubes for breakfast ever again and you may not ask me to.

5. When you want a snack between meals, you may help yourself to fresh fruit.

6. You may not tell your friends that we're ruining your life.

Encouragement is vital for success. If it's too hard to please you, a child will stop trying, but if reward always comes with reasonable effort, it's somewhat addictive. If you are going to insist on behavior change, the least you can do is pay attention and notice when they do what you want. Praise for every good decision and every good action will pay off in time.

Posting rules is a very important thing to do. Young children often respond very well to achievement charts. If your children are too young to read, you can draw a picture that represents each rule down the side of a piece of poster board and write the days of the week across the top. Every day they follow the rule, they can earn a star. If they get enough stars, take them to the park or let them pick an inexpensive toy from a grab bag you make up on a visit to the local dollar store. Young children can only handle a few rules at a time. Your child's age plus 1 is a maximum number to start with.

For older kids, and for yourself, a simple list on the fridge is generally sufficient, but rewards are important at every age. Choose a goal and plan to celebrate each achievement as a family.

It's almost impossible not to perceive some level of adversity in the effort it takes to eat healthy in the modern world, especially when you're first starting out, yet adversity binds people together. The up-side to this perception of adversity is the experience of teamwork it can facilitate between you and your older kids. Let them know this is hard for you, too, and that you need their help and encouragement. Let older kids participate in menu planning and teach them food preparation skills so they can be a real help. The extra togetherness and true quality time can be a huge blessing if you do it right.

Maybe one of your early goals is a short family trip where you prepare and pack all your food and don't buy anything while you're gone. It's a challenge you can all work together on, preparing and packing the food and planning where to go and what to do.

- Make it easy.

You want to change things, but it doesn't have to be hard to be successful. Do what you can to make it easy and fun for yourself as well as your kids. Here are a few suggestions for making healthy food friendly.

It's still all about marketing, so you need to be careful how you name the product. If I want my 7-year-old to have a healthy breakfast, I'm not going to suggest a Banana-Blueberry Bliss smoothie. I'm going to explain that we're going to try to eat really healthy this week because we don't like being sick. Then I'll ask her if she'd like some ice cream for breakfast. If I freeze the bananas and use very little coconut milk, this smoothie is so thick it looks, and feels, like ice cream—and it's blue! I'll serve it in a bowl with a spoon, let her sprinkle a little blueberry granola cereal on top, and everybody's happy.

Kids like ice cream and smoothies, once they learn to trust them. You can begin the process by relying more heavily on these tricks and transition to more veggies as they get more accustomed to healthy eating. Some of the transition happens quite naturally, because as they see you *enjoying* new things, their natural curiosity makes them want a taste. Don't worry if they make a face the first few times. This isn't an overnight process.

It's also possible to convert a lot of old favorites into new healthier versions. Spaghetti, chili, and pretty much any casserole can be changed to make it much healthier. Crumble up a product called tempeh instead of the usual ground beef. Try adding spinach chopped ultra fine or finely grated carrot to these sorts of dishes. If canned soup is involved, switch to a healthier variety without msg or other chemicals. Amy's is a good brand and there are others in the grocery health food section as well.

If your kids are used to canned vegetables and they won't touch fresh ones, try overcooking (not burning) the fresh ones a few times and backing off the cooking time little by little to help them adjust to the firmer texture.

Mix increasing amounts of whole grain pasta in with the white to ease that transition. This can work with rice, too, as long as you observe the difference in cooking times between whole grain and white.

Sometimes parents are more afraid of healthy food than kids are. We're afraid to offer some things because we fear the children will react badly. We shouldn't make assumptions, however. It's surprising what kids will eat and what they'll like sometimes when we don't prejudice them. Lay out a tray of fresh veggies or fruits and just see what they do. A child who pitches a fit about fresh cooked green beans might just like them raw.

• Where do you draw the line?

I try to respect my children's preferences within reason, especially as they get older. I draw a pretty hard line on what isn't allowed, but offer flexibility, and continuing education, as long as they stay on the right side of the fence. That means I don't allow the 4F foods in my house at all, but as long as they stay within the framework of fresh fruits, veggies, nuts, seeds, whole grains, beans etc I don't dictate too much. I don't say which veggies, which fruits, or how much. When you're doing what's right you should feel free.

The easiest way to make all this happen is to have no unhealthy choices in the house. That's how you manage temptation for yourself and your kids and it keeps you from feeling like the food police.

• New babies

If you have a new baby, you're in the best position of all. Babies are still forming their opinions of what tastes good. For better or worse, you set your baby's tastes by what you eat as well as by the foods you feed him. If you are nursing your baby, that's wonderful. You should continue for at least the duration of the first year. Continuing to nurse, as a supplement to a healthy diet, is a great thing throughout the second or even the third year. As you eat healthier food, you baby will learn to enjoy what's good for him through your milk.

I don't approve of cereals for babies less than one year old. Using cereals too early can lead to digestive inflammation and possible food allergies later on. Starting with non-citrus fruits and proceeding to vegetables is what I suggest, since fruits are easiest to digest. I don't like to begin solid foods at all before 5 or 6 months. One sign of readiness is the emergence of the first tooth, but if it comes at only two or three months, don't listen to it.

Some people are very nervous nursing their babies. If the baby seems hungry often, they assume he isn't getting enough or that milk is not enough for him. These assumptions are incorrect. Babies this age are growing rapidly and human milk is so easy for human babies to digest. They fill up, get what they need and are ready for more very soon. That's all perfectly normal. There will be days you feel that all you do is nurse your baby—that's perfectly normal, too. Don't be concerned, just feed him when he's hungry. The only reason bottle babies eat on a schedule is that formula is much more difficult to digest and so it takes longer. That's not a good thing. It's convenient, but not healthy.

Assuming it is time for solid food, when you make fresh veggies for yourself, put whatever is left over in the blender to make a puree. Freeze this in ice cube trays then seal it in labeled freezer bags so you have high quality baby food on demand. Just warm it and serve it. Foods that work well for this purpose include smoothies, individual fruits, broccoli, sweet potatoes, carrots, green beans, peas, and hard squashes.

Giving your baby fresh juices and smoothies in the baby bottle is also a great thing. When mine were toddlers, they drank a lot of smoothies. We split some nipples to allow the smoothies to flow and they took those everywhere. It's best to dilute vegetable juices and smoothies for babies under a year old. Start with half juice or smoothie and half water, just an ounce or two early on. By the time they are two, they should be able to handle 2–3 ounces of juice or 6 ounces of smoothie without any water added.

I'm ready. How do I get started?

You're mentally prepared. You know what to do and why you want to do it. How do you unleash all this enthusiasm in a productive way?

Begin by speaking with a few key friends and family members to assess what sort of support or opposition you will encounter. If your decision is worrisome to some of these key players in your life, it doesn't mean you can't or shouldn't proceed. Did they ask if their diet bothers you? It simply means that when you need support, you'll look for it somewhere else.

Involving friends and family as much as they are willing is wonderful and it can be a lot of fun, but if you have limited support among friends or family, you'll need to broaden your circle. It helps to work with a mentor or a specialist, especially if you have some major health challenges.

Contact me if you need me via my website at www.awesomehealthmakeover. com. You can read articles, watch videos, and listen to audios there. All of these are ways to increase your knowledge and support yourself emotionally. Eventually, I'll probably offer an online support group as well.

Creating a supportive environment is very important, too. Removing bad food is part of that process. You also need to keep a notebook or file box for simple recipes you like and ideas that worked for you. It's good to refer to this when you're feeling stuck and you need suggestions.

Posting reminders on the fridge and supportive "notes to self" in places you'll see regularly can be extremely helpful. Your standards and goals from chapter 1 should be among these notes.

There are several important lists and acronyms in this book that can help you remember critical information. I have compiled those at the end of the book in appendix A so you can write them down easily.

When your support is arranged, and your kitchen is ready, there's nothing left to do but—do it. Set up your salad box, dust off your blender and make some great healthy food. Enjoy!

Review

Key #6 Maximize Your Nutrition

You are what you eat.

Step one: Arrange your support system.

Step two: Make your environment supportive.

Step three: Get rid of non-foods, especially 4F foods.

Step four: Buy necessary equipment.

Step five: Re-stock your kitchen with healthy food.

Step six: Just do it!

Chapter 7: Exercise

This chapter is really about what I call body resource ecology. That means how your body uses what it has to continuously recreate your internal environment. Remember that in the introduction we mentioned the fact that, due to ongoing cell replacement, you grow an entirely new body every year or so. Whether good news or bad news, it isn't the same body each time. It's constantly changing. We talked about the fact that you are what you eat and absorb; those are your resources. But how those resources are arranged is determined by how you use your body. Remember, your body speaks body language. You tell it how to allocate resources every day. There are two principles that govern this process:

1. *Use it or lose it.* The "use it or lose it" principle applies most specifically to muscle and bone tissue—two key tissues that help keep you looking and feeling young and able. Have you ever seen what happens to an injured athlete's muscles? If a runner breaks a leg and wears a cast for several weeks, you see a big difference in his two legs when the cast comes off. Given his inability to exercise, both legs lose muscle, but the one that was totally immobilized loses far more, right? In this context we all understand the use it or lose it concept.

2. *You don't get what you don't ask for—managing your inner efficiency expert.* A similar principle applies to those who sit behind a desk all day or those who exercise only their remote control or texting finger. This principle states that

you will only build what your actions demand—you don't get anything you don't ask for.

Imagine that somewhere in the control center of your brain, there is a little balding man with black-rimmed glasses and a pocket protector keeping stats on which bones and muscles you use and how much you use them daily—your inner efficiency geek (IEG). It's his job to decide where to build more tissue and where to build less; you only have a finite amount of materials and energy to work with, after all. If you're the guy in the broken leg example, your inner expert will see that you aren't using your leg muscles much these days, so he'll shift resources away from those muscles. It's only sensible.

Let's assume you're a marginally healthy desk-jockey who has noticed his legs are looking flimsy while his muffin top is looming large, so you've started a new exercise routine. Your efficiency manager is excited. Things have changed and he has new numbers to work with. Here's what he's thinking: You did half an hour of light aerobics three times in 10 days and the result is that your leg muscles and lower back muscles are fatigued. Your IEG will now allocate additional resources to build up muscle tissue in your legs and low back.

This is how you put in a request for more muscle—by using your body. Your inner expert can see that you need more muscle, and more bone tissue, too, when you push your body out of its comfort zone. You tell your body what to build and where to build it by how you use it. You're speaking body language every minute of every day.

All of this is true whether you are a heavy weight contender, a newborn baby, or a paraplegic. Your body systems are the same. Every living thing depends on movement in so many ways. It's also true for your brain. Using your mind keeps your mind sharp. This is why people who are aging need mentally stimulating conversation and activity to help prevent mental degeneration.

Your lymphatic system—How movement helps

Have you ever sat too still for too long? You know that really stiff, stale feeling you get all over? When you don't get up and move your body, it feels like nothing is moving on the inside either, right? That's because when you move your muscles, you are moving your lymph fluid and nutrients and wastes are being transported to and from your cells. When you don't move, lymph fluid doesn't move. Cells don't get nutrients, including oxygen, and they don't get their trash picked up, at least not efficiently.

In chapter 5 we discussed the fact that you have a built-in pump—your heart, to move your blood around your body. But your blood doesn't carry nutrients in or wastes out at the cellular level. Your bloodstream is like the airlines—they are the major movers. They don't come to your door. You take a taxi to the airport where you get on the plane.

If your bloodstream is the airline, your lymph fluid is the local taxi service; but unlike your blood, your lymph fluid has no pump. It only moves when you move. Because of this need to move lymph fluid to cleanse and feed your cells, exercise greatly impacts your quality of life. How much?

You could rightly say that as you move, so shall you live. The difference between a person who exercises and one who doesn't is like the difference between a clean flowing stream and a stagnant pond. Which would you rather live in—literally?

Why movement is necessary—even in healthy tissue

Even in healthy tissue, each cell produces waste products that need to be removed. It's just natural. Every scientist knows that two requirements for keeping cells alive in a dish are that you must continually remove waste and continually feed the cells what they need. Failure to remove waste will cause an alteration in the pH of the dish. If the pH changes much at all, the cells will die.

Cells inside your body are no different. They can continue to live and function only within a certain pH range. Outside that range, death is immediate. Even bacterial cells work this way. One of the methods of killing germs on household surfaces is to use products that are acidic to create a harsh environment to kill the bacteria. When we create harsh terrain in the body, cells die or become cancerous.

Specific benefits of exercise

You can see that exercise directly benefits every cell in your body. The relationship between movement and cellular benefit is direct and immediate; like turning the crank on a music box to hear the music play faster. As your movement increases, your cells get faster service

You can't feel your cells saying "ahhhh" when you move around, but you can feel the effect when large numbers of cells become healthier. Large clusters of cells of the same type are called tissues. Tissues make up organs. Organs functioning optimally keep you running and feeling healthy. At this level, we can really quantify the benefits of exercise in your life.

• Movement helps you heal and recover from illness or injury.

Because of the role of movement in removing wastes and bringing nutrients to your cells, movement is critical for healing anything. There is no injury or disease that will not be improved at least on some level when exercise of some sort is part of your routine.

You know that if you cut your finger, you need to keep the wound clean to help it heal. Tissues inside the body are no different. They all need to be kept clean and well-fed in order to facilitate healing.

When a tissue is damaged, individual cells are injured and their contents are spilled into the surrounding fluid. This creates a toxic environment for the remaining cells whose job it will be to replace those which have been destroyed. Movement helps flush these toxins away from the site to improve the healing capacity by creating a more cell-friendly environment.

Even though serious medical conditions will usually prevent vigorous exercise, movement is critical to help you recover. There is no way to heal any tissue in your body as long as it is starved for nutrients and bathed in toxic waste.

As discussed in chapter 5, the closest thing to a pump for your lymph fluid is your diaphragm. Even the sickest person is still breathing, and how you breathe matters. Making the most of this simplest of exercises can go a long way toward improving your health in the worst of circumstances.

Not only does the mechanical aspect of breathing help feed and cleanse your cells, but the body language aspect of correct diaphragmatic breathing calms the mind and puts the nervous system in the right mode for healing. Like any other exercise, breathing can be improved and gradually increased to improve your health.

Fortunately, even a little bit of movement makes a big difference—and that's really good news for the critically ill as well as the chronologically challenged. You don't have to run a marathon to be well, you just have to keep moving.

- Got energy?

Everything that happens in your body obeys those two functional principles; use it or lose it, and you don't get what you don't ask for. Energy is produced based on assessed need. Your inner efficiency geek determines today's energy output based on yesterday's demand. If you are sedentary, you will produce less energy every hour of the day than someone who is active. Think of all the ramifications of this concept.

It's not oversimplified to say that getting some exercise first thing in the morning sets your energy factory at a higher gear for the whole day. If you are producing more energy all day long, you not only have enough to get through your morning jog, but also enough to get through that afternoon meeting without dozing off. You're also burning more calories per hour—all day long. That's a great thing if you are trying to lose weight or keep it off.

- Weight Control

Exercise is absolutely essential for weight loss. Anyone who tells you that permanent weight loss without exercise is possible is either delusional or he's trying to sell you a miracle pill. The use-it-or-lose-it principle has to be modified for weight loss. Here, it's use it *TO* lose it!

This is another area where your own common sense is your best defense. What determines your weight? At its simplest level, weight is *determined* by the number of calories you take in *beyond what you can burn immediately*. Obviously, there are two factors within your control in this equation—what you take in, and how much you burn. The bottom line, mathematically speaking, is that if you are already overweight and you want to shed pounds, you must bring in fewer calories than you need to burn—at every hour of the day—so that you are always burning stored fuel (fat).

If you eat next to nothing all day long, then have a big meal at the end of the day, you will still add fat. Why? Because in that one meal, which is occurring at a time when your metabolism is about to slow down for the day, you are taking in more calories than you will be able to burn before you go to bed. Those extra calories, in that very hour, will be converted to fat. There is no way around that. It's like gravity, it applies to everyone.

As we mentioned before, getting exercise in the morning sets you up to burn more calories all day long. Additionally, the muscles you build by exercising more will help you achieve your weight loss goals.

Muscles burn calories—even when they aren't being used. Fat cells never do any work, so they never use many calories. It's the difference between feeding a barn-full of racehorses and a barn-full of feeder pigs. They take up similar amounts of barn space, but the racehorses eat a whole lot more, even on the days you don't run them. For weight control purposes, you want your barn full of the finest thoroughbreds broccoli and spinach can buy.

Yet another good reason to swap those fat cells for muscle cells, fat cells can be used as storage for harmful toxins far more easily than muscle cells. You don't need to store toxins, you need to get rid of them. Being overweight creates extra work for your entire body including your liver and kidneys which are responsible for removing the toxins from your body. Unburdening your liver and kidneys helps you process the toxins instead of storing them.

My final pitch for losing weight: fat cells actually produce estrogen. Yes, men, even *your* fat cells do it. Because you are entirely a hormonally driven being, hormonal imbalance increases your risk for every disease. *Every single one.* In cancer, heart disease, and diabetes, the effects of excess estrogen are fairly well understood.

Estrogen makes things grow—which is the last thing you want if you have cancer. Excess estrogen also has a negative impact of the effectiveness of insulin; not very helpful if you are diabetic. The classic picture of heart disease risk is the man with a lot of belly fat—belly fat makes a lot of excess estrogen. Estrogen tends to make inflammation worse—and this includes the inflammation in your arteries which leads to heart disease.

- Vascular health

Speaking of heart disease, did you know that even your blood vessels have muscle? Blood vessel walls are muscular, that's how they can expand and contract to influence your blood pressure on demand. These muscles need to be worked just like any others, and these tissues respond to improvements in your diet and exercise habits more quickly than most.

Because they are in such close contact with your blood supply, blood vessel cells get first dibs on all the nutrients and cleansing your body can provide. This is great news for those who have heart disease. If you have heart disease and you want to delve into this subject more deeply, I recommend reading *Dr. Dean Ornish's Program for Reversing Heart Disease: The Only System Scientifically Proven to Reverse Heart Disease Without Drugs or Surgery.*

- Brain function and stress handling

When you have established an exercise program and you are producing more energy, your mind functions better. When your mind is sharp you handle everything more easily and so you have less tendency to feel overwhelmed and stressed. This is one very important tool in managing key #1—attitude.

When you exercise, your body also produces endorphins. Endorphins are chemicals that increase your sense of happiness and well-being. Many people have found that regular exercise works as well as any anti-depressant. That alone is a great reason to work it into your schedule.

Even the ability to resist the mental declines associated with aging is related to exercise. It's been discovered that, because the mind-body connection is strengthened by exercise, mental faculties such as memory and reasoning skills are improved and retained later in life by those who continue to get regular exercise.

Based on the use-it-or-lose-it principle, elderly folk who remain active also tend to have better reflexes and better balance. Improved reflexes and balance go a long way toward preventing those debilitating falls that result in broken arms and hips among the elderly.

- Exercise doesn't work for me...

On a side note, there are people for whom this doesn't seem to work. If exercising makes you feel run-down and you just can't get used to it, you probably have low functioning adrenal and thyroid glands. This is the very reason exercise is the last of the 7 Keys. If you work through the other six, it gives your body time to heal a bit and build up some reserve before you demand more from it.

What kind of exercise is best?

There are basically three types of exercise; cardiovascular, strength training, and stretching. Examples of these would include running, weight lifting, and yoga respectively. Now that you are totally convinced you need to get some exercise, how do you decide what to do? We'll look at each type and see what considerations you need to take into account.

1. Cardiovascular

Exercises aimed at building up your heart and lungs are referred to as cardiovascular, or just cardio for short. There are lots of activities that qualify including tennis, racquetball, aerobics, jogging, cycling, swimming, hiking, walking, you get the idea—constant motion of your whole body.

Everybody needs some cardiovascular exercise. This is probably the best choice when you want to boost your energy production, burn calories, or improve your heart health. It's also the one people are most likely to overdo. While people were made for sustained activity and we are dependent on constant movement to feed and clean our cells, we weren't really well designed to go all out for very long.

It is increasingly well-established that mild cardiovascular exercise, such as walking, conveys as much health benefit, and in some cases more benefit, than running or heavy-duty aerobics. People who engage in excessive activities— repeatedly running marathons or obsessive aerobics devotees—ultimately develop scarring in the heart which can interfere with heart function.

Consistent low-level activity with occasional bursts of intensity such as occurs when you are gardening, cleaning your house, or taking a walk after dinner with your significant other are ideal for meeting human needs for movement. There's nothing wrong with preparing for and running a 5k either, but don't think that you have to go that far to get the benefits cardiovascular exercise provides. The more time you spend on your feet, the better—regardless of what you're doing.

2. Strength training, weight-bearing exercise

Once again, everybody needs some strength training exercises to maintain optimal health. Basically, this means weight-bearing exercise. It can be done with resistance equipment, with free weights, or even isometrically, but the theme here is to isolate a major muscle group and stress it—a lot.

Strength training builds muscle and keeps bones strong due to the two principles of use it or lose it and you don't get what you don't ask for. The benefits of more muscle and bone are obvious. If you have very little muscle, even a small job may be enough to push your muscles, ligaments, or tendons to the point of injury. If your muscles are bigger and stronger however, every job you do is far less of a strain.

• Injury prevention

Building core muscle strength in your abdomen and your back is the best way to prevent back strain, tension headaches, and other muscle related soreness. Being strong physically is also a good way to prevent dangerous falls because you'll have more strength and balance to compensate for the unexpected. More muscle = less chance of injury and less strain and pain from normal daily activity.

• Best exercise for diabetics

Strength training is a great asset for the diabetic. Because muscle cells burn more sugar, and store more sugar, than fat cells, having more muscle means better blood sugar control.

• Very important in osteoporosis

As we discussed before, when it comes to building your body, you don't get what you don't ask for. The two biggest reasons people succumb to osteoporosis are lack of weight bearing exercise, and hormonal imbalance. Improper diet (too much animal-sourced protein, not enough nutrients) is a very close inter-related third, and inadequate calcium supplementation doesn't even make the list.

3. Simple static isometrics to get you started

Some of the best things in life are free, especially where exercise is concerned. Simple push-ups are hard to beat for back and upper body strength, but they aren't safe for everyone and too many of them can cause joint problems. This is true for all weight-bearing exercises. They're good for muscles and bones, but very hard on joints.

The way to have the best of both worlds is to start with static isometrics, if you're a beginner, or something called Static Contraction if you're already reasonably fit.

Static isometrics are easy and cost nothing. Safer for children who are too young for weights, and much safer for anyone who has to exercise alone, isometric exercises involve only the weight of your own body. Taking the push-up example, which can cause damage to your shoulder joints over time, just try doing one push-up—for as long as you can hold it half-way down.

By only going through the range of motion once, you spare your joints, but by holding up your body weight for a prolonged period, you stress your arm bones and muscles. This method has proven to build more muscle in a shorter period of time with fewer workouts than any traditional free-weight or resistance program.

The key difference between static and conventional strength training is this: In static isometrics or static contraction, you make progress by increasing the duration of a single repetition of each exercise and/or by increasing the weight during a single repetition. In conventional strength training, you progress by increasing the number of repetitions and/or the weight.

Almost any conventional calisthenic exercise can be converted to a static isometric exercise by going halfway through it and holding your position. Static Contraction exercises—for the more advanced among us—operate on the same principle by holding a free weight in a specified position. You can't do this however, without more information, proper equipment, and one or two partners to keep you from dropping the weights on yourself. For more information on this excellent strength-training program by Pete Sisco, go to www.precisiontraining.com.

4. Stretching

There are various disciplines of stretching exercises that are very beneficial, some steeped in tradition and culture, others strictly practical. Of those with cultural depth, tai chi and yoga are probably the most widely practiced. Apart from these, most stretching programs are either used before or after some other athletic pursuit or they may be designed to address a very particular condition such as pregnancy or a strained muscle.

It really doesn't at all do justice to yoga or tai chi to refer to them as stretching exercises. I designate them as such because it is the flexibility and range of motion they offer that distinguishes them from cardiovascular or strength training. But while strength training and cardiovascular exercises don't offer much flexibility and range of motion, yoga and tai chi do assist with cardiovascular fitness and strength.

If you wanted to practice one discipline which would give you a well-rounded exercise experience, yoga or tai chi would most closely fill the bill. There are several different forms of yoga and tai chi and there are clear differences among them. Some are much more intensive than others, building more strength and stamina, while some are far less intense, focused more on flexibility and energy balance. Beginner levels of these arts are, of course, lower impact than more advanced levels.

Yet another dimension of yoga and tai chi is the energetic balance they can help to maintain or restore. While many exercises focus more on one side of the body or one limb, yoga and tai chi attempt to give equal attention to all parts of the body to create a much more balanced muscle tone throughout the body. This is a very good feature since lack of symmetry can lead to spinal misalignments that contribute to many other health complaints.

All forms of stretching help you lengthen and relax tense muscles which can reduce the chance for injury. Sore muscles have an excessive concentration of lactic acid which stretching can help to reduce. Even the muscular aspect of the arteries benefit from stretching.

Many back and shoulder problems can be improved with a properly applied and well-balanced program of stretching. If you have a significant problem of long-standing, a physical therapist or chiropractor should be consulted before you begin any serious stretching.

Start where you are

Each person has unique exercise needs. The first step toward meeting your needs is to find your starting point by assessing your present condition. Whether you are already a top-notch athlete or you are bed-ridden, there are things you can do, and things you can do better.

Maybe as an athlete your focus has been on cardio and strength, but you haven't really taken stretching to the next level. Maybe you're a couch potato and you just need to get up and start something. After reading here about these three types of movement you need to address, you should think about simple ways to include all three in your exercise program.

The greatest value of accurately assessing your condition lies in your ability to avoid overdoing it. The most common mistake people make when trying to start exercising is being too ambitious not only in type, but also in quantity of exercise. Pain and exhaustion will kill your motivation before you even make a good start.

Have you ever done the weekend warrior routine, taking on a heavy project or activity you aren't used to? You don't just feel sore for an hour or two. Recovery takes several days—the effect is cumulative. If walking a mile is something you know you could do today, don't. Remember that the effects of exercise are cumulative over several days, and your body isn't used to the added energy demands you're about to make. Start well below your maximum capacity, then slowly and consistently increase your speed, time, and distance.

If you aren't already involved in a sport or an exercise program, I highly recommend that your first step be to build on your present activity level. There are lots of small ways to do this without turning your life upside down.

Make small lifestyle adjustments first

The most important thing you can do is to keep this simple at the start. Don't sign up for a gym membership you'll be too uncomfortable to use, don't buy expensive equipment you'll never find the time to learn how to assemble, and don't download step-by-step instructions from internet exercise gurus no one else has ever heard of. This doesn't have to be hard and it doesn't have to change who you are.

Think of exercise in terms of movement. Every movement counts. Make your world more movement centered and become more aware of opportunities for movement throughout your day. Here are some simple suggestions:

- Take the stairs instead of the elevator.
- Become a far-parker.
- Take a walk after dinner with your family.
- Play some music at your desk that will keep you tapping your feet.
- Take a break every 30 minutes for 1 minute of stretching and 1 minute of deep breathing.
- Get off the couch, move the couch, and learn to dance with your spouse instead of just watching TV every evening.
- Get a big rubber exercise ball. Sit on that instead of the couch and bounce during your favorite show.

These are little things but they add up to a more active lifestyle. It's really not about what you do for 30 minutes twice each week—that's not enough. It's about what you do all day long and how you do it.

Make the most of what you already do

It may help you to keep an exercise journal for a week. Write down what you are already doing physically. Do you go to the grocery store or a discount store where you have to walk a lot? Do you have stairs in your house? Do you have a garden? Do you have a friend, or an eager dog, who keeps asking you to walk with her in the mornings? Do you clean your house over the weekend? Do you play golf? See what you've got to work with and think about how to build on those assets.

You can walk every aisle in the store instead of just a few. Back up and repeat the middle few steps each time you go up or down the stairs. Refurbish your garden. Say yes to your friend, at least occasionally. Play some catchy music that really gets you moving while you clean the house. Walk the first 9 instead of driving the cart for all 18 holes.

Apart from simply increasing the level of activities you already do, one of the easiest and most effective ways to introduce more cardio gently into your life is simply to take a little walk each day. Your present level of fitness will determine whether that walk is around the house, around the block, or an extra turn around the grocery store, but what matters is that you take whatever the next step is for you—every day.

Going to the next level with cardio and more

While it's true that a journey of a thousand miles begins with the next step, don't plan a thousand mile hike as your next step. Remember that the next step is just that—one single action, not a life-altering event.

For cardio exercise, regardless of what sport or activity you choose, it would be better to start out at about 1/3 of your total capacity and do it several times through the week. After the first week, you'll have a better idea of how it will cumulatively affect you and your body will begin to adjust to a higher energy output to support your effort.

The top three forms of cardio exercise, in order, are: rebounding, swimming in non-chlorinated water, and walking or hiking. If you choose to rebound, make sure you get a good mini-trampoline. Good ones are tight enough to prevent your ankles from rolling in every time you come down. Consistently rolling your ankles can cause misalignment in your spine.

Choose your activity, assess your starting point, set a goal, and build up to it slowly. If you have a serious medical condition or a handicap, you will need to get professional help to design a safe and suitable plan tailored to meet your needs and prevent injury.

Take your flexibility to the next level with stretching

If you participate in any kind of sport, you probably already do a little basic stretching when you play. Many people don't realize that stretching is not as safe or beneficial when your muscles are cold. If you walk or jog, for example, it's best to walk a few minutes, stop and stretch, then do the bulk of your work out. Stretching cold muscles can cause damage or cramping because your circulation isn't moving enough. If you're going to do more serious stretching, it's better to do it after your workout than before.

For a more intensive flexibility program, it's hard to beat yoga. There are lots of yoga and tai chi instructional videos to get you started—and they're free! Most public libraries carry several you could try. Just be careful you don't start with something too advanced for your level. There are also classes at the local YMCA/YWCA, at many gyms, and of course by private instruction if you are ready to go that far.

Yoga and tai chi are initially focused on flexibility and balance at the beginner level. As you move into intermediate or advanced techniques, strength and cardiovascular fitness are involved also for a very thorough approach to your exercise needs.

There are simple ways to get started with stretching on your own. One of the most basic stretching exercises is touching your toes (or trying to). It's easier, and safer, for most people to do this sitting down. If you really can't even get close, it may help you to work with a strap. An old belt, a piece of rope, or your dog's leash can be placed under one foot at a time. Hold the ends of the strap and pull gently.

The toe touch lengthens your low-back muscles and your leg muscles, which is helpful for the millions who cope with low-back and hip pain. It's really good for everyone. You probably get more bang for your buck out of this one stretch than any other.

Another area worth working on is your chest. Many people feel back discomfort and try to stretch their back muscles when the real problem is tightness through the chest, which draws the shoulders forward. If you place your hands on either side of a doorway in your house and then move forward gently, you will feel a good stretch through your chest and upper arms. Try this with your hands at various heights on the door frame.

The biggest problem with stretching, like cardio, is overdoing it. While there is some truth to the "no pain, no gain" idea, there is a big difference between mild discomfort and agony. If the pain is too great, you will be unable to relax the muscle you are trying to stretch. Bracing and resisting will largely negate the benefits of any stretching exercise.

Here are five things to remember when stretching:
1. Get your circulation going and warm up your muscles a little before stretching.

2. Relax the muscle you're stretching.
3. Don't hold the stretch too long or do it too hard. Be gentle.
4. Don't "bounce."
5. Don't forget to breathe.

If you work on your lower back and legs, and your chest, each day for even a few minutes, you'll soon begin to feel a difference.

Do-it-yourself strength training

It's a good idea to start with cardio and flexibility exercises first, then move on to strength training when you've already established your exercise habit. This is because while cardio and stretching exercises need to be done consistently and often to be most effective, strength training works best when it isn't overdone. I recommend strength training once every week to ten days and alternate cardio and stretching in between.

A typical week might look like this:

Monday:	Take a walk after dinner for 30 minutes.
Tuesday:	Do a 20-minute yoga video with a friend.
Wednesday:	Walk during your lunch hour for 30 minutes.
Thursday:	Do the 20-minute yoga video again.
Friday:	Walk 30 minutes.
Saturday:	20-minute strength training using static isometric exercises.
Sunday:	Rest.

For safety's sake, you really should walk for a few minutes or do something else to warm up your muscles before you do any stretching or strength-training exercises, and you should stretch out again afterward. Strength-training days really include all three types of exercises.

If you are starting from square zero, you could begin with the most basic of all—push-ups and sit-ups. Get a watch and a pencil and paper to record what sort of exercises you'll try and what your times were for each one. From the classic push-up position, lower yourself halfway to the ground and then stop. Count the seconds and see how long you can hold the position before your arms are shaky and about to give out. Follow the same routine with the sit-ups and with any other exercise you can go half-way through and stop. Squats and pull-ups work pretty well. Write down what you do and how many seconds you manage to hold each position.

That's your baseline. Next week, when you're fully recovered, you can try to break your records.

It might take up to a week to get beyond the soreness and fully recover from this sort of exercise, which is normal, so wait that long before you try it again. Muscle is built during the recovery period between exercises, while you are healing, not during the actual workout, so you never want to short-change your recovery period. Each time, you should be able to hold each position a little longer. If you can't, you likely need more recovery time between exercise sessions.

You can do a five minute warm-up walk, 10 minute exercise session (4-6 different exercises), and 5 minutes of stretching afterward for a total of just 20 minutes. As a raw beginner, you only need to do this once every week to ten days to meet your specific strength-building needs—not a bad deal! This plan won't help you win a body-builder contest any time soon, but it's a good first step.

Thinking beyond the next step, it's also good to have a bigger goal—something to look forward to. Maybe you've always wanted to learn to play tennis but you don't have the stamina. If so, you'll be walking or climbing those stairs with purpose—to build up enough strength to take a few tennis lessons. Having a goal ahead helps you stay motivated. There are endless possibilities—mountain climbing, horseback riding, skiing, roller skating, whatever suits your taste. It's all good.

How to move when confined to your bed or chair

If you really are bedridden or wheelchair bound, you'll have to think much smaller for now, but don't fall into the trap of thinking that what little you can do won't matter. It will. Here is a short list of simple movements most people can do even from the bed, chair—or desk. Don't worry about the things on this list you can't do, just focus on what you can.

If your health is so poor that you can't be up and about, you definitely need to be pushing the envelope of your abilities, in safe ways, every day. As we discussed before, never allow yourself to think that what you are able to do is so small it won't matter. It will help. Here are a few simple movements you can make to get lymph flowing without leaving your bed or chair:

- Tighten and release your calf muscles. This is far more beneficial than you might imagine. Military personnel sometimes use this exercise to boost circulation when they have to stand for long periods of time. It can assist your circulation as well which would surely be a very good thing while your larger movements are limited.

- Lift your legs or move them side to side. Make circles. These movements strengthen your lower back and abdominal muscles.

- Lying flat on your back with your arms stretched out to your sides, draw your knees up toward your chest. Allow your bent knees and your lower body to gently roll to one side then the other while keeping both shoulders flat against the bed. This helps to stretch your lower back.

- Roll your neck forward and from side to side very slowly and gently if you are sitting up. If you must lie down, just turn your head from side to side.

- Tighten and release your arm muscles and your hands.

- Raise you leg a bit and make a circular motion with your foot.

- Bend your knees and straighten them.

- Move your arms up and down and from side to side.

- Make circles with your arms.

- For total body stress reduction and relaxation, try to progressively tighten every muscle you have control of from your toes to the top of your head. Hold them tight for a couple of seconds, then release. This helps re-teach your body what it feels like to really relax.

Basically anything will help. Just move!

If you can't move at all

Movement works even when you can't do it by yourself. Having someone else move your arms and legs for you still provides the lymphatic movement necessary to help you cleanse and feed your tissues. Massage accomplishes this goal also. There is a very light and superficial lymphatic massage which focuses on moving lymph fluid for you, and there is also deeper more intense massage focusing on moving the acids out of muscle tissues. All these therapies are extremely beneficial and should be provided for those who cannot move sufficiently on their own.

The final analysis

The ultimate question of which type of exercise is best has not one answer but three. All the evidence suggests that moderate exercise is generally best, that everyone can benefit from some level of exercise, and that each person really needs some of each of these three major types of exercise on an ongoing basis.

Maybe you've heard the expression, "If you pick up a calf every day, you can lift it when it's a cow." That may not be true, but this is: whatever you want to be able to do when you're 80, you'd better be doing triple that when you're 40. Use it, or lose it.

Review

Key #7 Exercise

As you move, so shall you live.

Step one: Assess your fitness level. Get professional help if necessary.

Step two: Use an exercise journal to record how you move through a typical week and think of ways to build on that. Don't overdo it!.

Step three: Plan ways to include more cardio exercise in your life.

Step four: Plan ways to include more stretching in your life.

Step five: Plan ways to include some basic strength training in your life.

Chapter 8: Putting It All Together:

The Synergy of the 7 Keys

The word synergy means that some things are only amazing when you put them all together—they work together. Have you ever heard people singing in harmony? Each part alone sounds very ordinary, but when you put them all together, the sound can be stunningly beautiful. People take classes called "music appreciation" to help them fully appreciate all that went into making beautiful music. This is the health appreciation chapter. It's purpose is to help you fully experience the symphony of health through the harmony of all 7 Keys.

Now that you know a lot about each of the 7 Keys individually, we can talk about how they work together and assist each other in enhancing your health. They really don't so much enhance your health; they *are* your health process in action.

This synergy is important to grasp for three reasons. First, it is highly motivational when you have depth of knowledge combined with a high level understanding of health. Second it helps you make sense of the latest things you hear from friends or news sources. Third, it helps you see through short-sighted programs from "experts" who don't see the big picture. The big picture is your intellectual safety net just as the synergy of the 7 Keys is your physical one.

What do you hear from friends and neighbors? Maybe it's a buddy who says he doesn't think diet matters so much. After wasting years on one diet after another, he started a really great exercise program a few months ago and he's finally lost all the weight he needed to lose plus he feels and looks fantastic. He says forget diet, exercise is where it's at.

Maybe your cousin says just the opposite. She tried every exercise program out there and all of them just left her feeling drained. She only feels better when she takes these super vitamins, and she thinks everyone should have them.

Maybe you've got a doctor friend who is passionate about one of these 7 Keys, but ignores the others entirely. Have you noticed that the book stores are full of books on nutrition, books on exercise, books on stress management, but this is the only one that gives you ALL 7 Keys? Why?

Most people get very excited when they find something that makes sense, that works for them. They're so excited, they immediately stop looking for anything more. That's tragic! Have you ever seen someone adopt a vegetarian diet and try to convert everyone else only to decide five years later that he was wrong and it doesn't work long term? Why did that happen? This chapter answers those questions. You'll see why this program works—for life!

Biochemical individuality

The simplest answer to the question above is that everybody's different. Some people take that to mean that some should eat meat, while veggies are better for others. That's not accurate. While some do need more of certain vitamins or minerals than others do, some need more sleep than others, and some can tolerate more stress than others, we do all need the same things, we just need them in varying quantities.

Your buddy who did well with the exercise program has different needs within these 7 key categories than your cousin who took her vitamins—but they still have the same 7 key categories to work with. One key may carry more weight for one person than for another, but we all must address all 7 to be healthy for a lifetime. Every person's health status is like this bar graph of the 7 Keys based on their current needs or their performance. Notice that ideal for

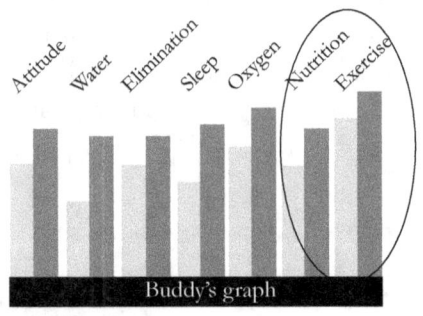
Buddy's graph

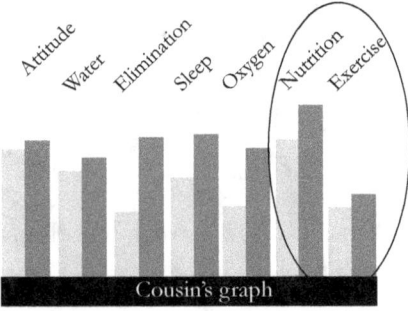
Cousin's graph

one isn't ideal for the other, but each one has the same 7 key areas.

Weakness in one area affects the others in different ways. Each combination of factors is unique.

Your buddy would surely get a lot more out of his exercise program if he also improved his diet, got more sleep, and managed his stress better, but he was so sedentary to start with that no diet alone would ever have reduced his weight sufficiently.

Your cousin could have gotten her vitamin needs met better by juicing and improving her diet. Once her nutritional needs were met, and she was sleeping better, she would surely benefit from the right sort of exercise also, but until she improved her nutritional status, she couldn't tolerate the exercise.

People tend to jump from one key to another—trying one or two at a time—and thinking they don't work. Finally, they hit on their weakest link and think they've found "the" answer.

That's a point worth repeating. Whenever someone believes he's found "the answer," what he's really found is his own weakest link. Your greatest potential for health challenges lies in whatever area your poorest performance intersects your highest need.

The problem is that today's weakest link won't necessarily be your weakest link ten years from now. You need a broad spectrum approach to get through a lifetime of health challenges.

How about the diet experts? There are lots of different ideas, but how many of them follow your physiology? How many account for your innate design? They frequently take their authority from what works in a chemistry lab, what comes out right on paper, or what works for lab rats, but that thinking never takes the current human equation into account. You have design issues (chapter 6) that have to be respected, and failure to work within those guidelines dooms one to eventual failure. Your body may be able to compensate to make it work for a little while, but not forever.

Some base their dietary recommendations on where they believe life originated and how they believe mankind evolved. Is it logical to base your assessment of your needs today on what some caveman supposedly ate a billion years ago? You don't need a working theory for the origin of mankind to know what you need to eat today. You need a working knowledge of how you are put together, right now. Your body is what it is today—and you can't change or evolve beyond that in your lifetime. You have to work with, and respect, what you have right now, regardless of how it got here.

Here's the secret to understanding why so many radically different approaches to diet work in some cases and not in others. The typical American diet is *SO bad*; nearly every fad diet out there is an improvement for most people. If nothing else, fad diets bring some variety into the nutritional wasteland most people call home, so they do feel some better at least for some time. Most all diet programs do get people away, at least temporarily, from processed food and that is a huge step in the right direction for most people.

What's the long-term answer? 7 Key Synergy; plain and simple. The rest of this chapter is about how the 7 keys work together to make your health as good as it can be. We'll look at it from several angles to fully appreciate the inter-relationships among all 7 keys, beginning with the fundamentals of the biochemistry of life.

That sounded complicated, but it isn't really. When you study chemistry and biology, you learn that life depends on millions of chemical reactions taking place in your body. Think of these reactions as plays in a game where your body is the field and the outcome is your life. All the plays are run by the same few players. They are oxygen, energy (fuel), and cofactors (nutrients).

Fuel is the quarterback, nutrients are all the other players, and oxygen is the ball. One team is called acid and the other team is called alkaline.

You run plays all day and all night. Sometimes acid wins, sometimes alkaline. If you don't take in any fuel—that's food, the quarterback gets sacked and you take a time out.

If the other players don't show up, it's really hard for the quarterback to complete a pass or for either team to score at all.

If the ball is missing, you don't play. The ball is required for every play just as oxygen is required for virtually all normal functions in the human body. It's not just breathing, it's chemistry. Processing food, making energy, and removing toxins are what life is about at it's most fundamental level. Those three functions are all about chemical reactions which all require oxygen.

That's the simplest analogy I can think of to give you a memorable framework to hang on to for the rest of this chapter. Let's look at how the 7 keys work together to support each other from several different perspectives.

The Oxygen Perspective on the 7 Keys

It's the insignificant-sounding one in the middle of the acronym. The one nobody ever writes a book about. Who needs to? We all breathe automatically and oxygen is everywhere. This one takes care of itself, right? If you already read chapter 5, you know it's not that simple.

Starting from the top, what relationship does attitude have with oxygen? When your oxygen is low, you are more likely to feel panic or depression. Handling stress becomes more difficult because your thinking is not as clear.

Due to the feedback cycle that exists with your adrenal glands, when you feel stressed, you are more likely to engage in shallow chest breathing which perpetuates the reduced oxygen problem in your body.

What about water? How does water relate to oxygen? H2O. There is oxygen in your water—it's one source. If you are dehydrated, you are also, by default, oxygen deficient. You can't fix one without the other, because remember that the bloodstream and lymph system you rely on to carry oxygen to your cells is mostly made up of water. It's hard to oxygenate properly without water as a source as well as a supply line.

How about elimination? Remember that I mentioned that pop and other caffeine sources increase your need for water, and we just discussed the relationship between dehydration and low oxygen. Furthermore, you eliminate things largely because they are toxins to your body. How do you get rid of toxins? Your body neutralizes toxins through lots of chemical reactions involving—yep, oxygen. You don't want to use up your oxygen just to clear your system of toxins. What a waste!

Next comes sleep. Surely that could have little to do with oxygen. As it happens, the quality of your sleep is definitely connected to your oxygen supply because of the relationship with stress handling. Low oxygen people are stressed out panic-prone people because shallow breathing tells the adrenal glands you aren't safe. People who are in perpetual stress response don't typically sleep well. Adrenal hormone cycles control how you sleep, and stress negatively impacts adrenal hormone balance. In turn, people who don't get good sleep don't repair their bodies properly and generate a lot of extra acids that have to be handled. Acid environments favor hydrogen, not oxygen. Increasing the acid level in your body further reduces the oxygen available for the reactions that keep you going strong.

Skipping oxygen itself in the acronym, we come to maximizing your nutrition. This one's big. Foods are generally categorized by content as proteins, fats, or carbohydrates, but they all have one thing in common. Proteins, fats and carbs are all made of things like nitrogen, carbon, and - oxygen. Complex carbohydrates have the most oxygen content by far of these three categories. That means fruits and veggies win big when you need to oxygenate your body. Since cooking releases a lot of the water content from fruits and veggies, raw ones have more oxygen to offer you than cooked ones.

How does exercise relate to oxygen? As you move, so shall you circulate, feed, and cleanse your body. Movement circulates the lymph fluids that carry all nutrients—including oxygen—to your cells. When you exercise, you also increase and deepen your breathing pattern to bring in more oxygen to your body.

Are you beginning to gain some appreciation for the synergy of the 7 keys? Let's repeat this exercise from the perspective of exercise.

The exercise perspective on 7 Key synergy

Exercise impacts attitude profoundly. Many people have proven for themselves that exercise stimulates endorphins which lift your spirits and improve your mood. Exercise has proven itself as effective as antidepressants and anti-anxiety medications time and again. Because it reduces anxiety and alleviates depression, it also improves the quality of your sleep. When you sleep better, you also have more energy for exercise. It's a great cycle.

Water intake tends to be higher among people who exercise for obvious reasons. You get hot and sweaty and that makes you thirsty. Good deal.

Elimination is greatly enhanced by exercise—elimination of bad habits, but also the other kind of elimination. Exercise is a good constipation cure—especially when you're drinking a lot of water! Drinking extra water also benefits you by keeping your kidneys flushed.

We already covered how exercise helps you sleep, but one distal concept we didn't mention here was the "use it or lose it" principle of body ecology. Your body builds tissues better while you sleep and it only builds what you put in a requisition for. If you lie around all day, you can expect losses in bone and muscle mass—you're telling your body you don't need resources there. As we discussed in chapter 7, stressing your bones and muscles tells your body to build up those tissues. Exercise, especially weight bearing exercise, is how you talk to your body about resource allocation.

Oxygen intake is increased when we exercise because we breathe hard and it is circulated better because we're moving our muscles.

Exercise improves nutrition partly because most people who bother to exercise think twice before they eat junk. When you are investing in your body in one way, you try a little harder in other areas, too. Exercise also is required to carry nutrients to those hard to reach places in the body. As you move so shall you...

So you can see how exercise works synergistically with the other keys to keep you well.

The maximum nutrition perspective on 7 Key synergy

One more round. How does nutrition give an assist to the other six keys? Nutrition helps your stress handling system very directly. Your nervous system requires a wide variety of B vitamins and minerals, for example, to keep you on an even keel. Lack of these cofactors can cause all sorts of psychological issues such as anxiety, depression, and reduced ability to cope with stress. Proportionately, the brain probably uses more nutrients than any other organ on a day to day basis—especially when we're under stress.

How does nutrition help with water? Of all the food you could eat, fruits and veggies are the biggest water contributors and, not surprisingly, they are the richest sources of nutrition in our diet. Most fruits and veggies are more than 50% water; and it's high quality water loaded with trace minerals. Obviously, if you juice your veggies, you get enormous bang for your buck. There is no better source of water, and no better multivitamin than a glass of freshly extracted vegetable juice.

As for elimination, excellent nutrition is the natural opposite of much of what you need to eliminate. If you are eating all the right things, there won't be much room for anything bad. Eating right helps people feel well, mentally and physically. When you are coping well, you are also better able to tackle non-food items that should be eliminated as well. Hopefully not literally.

Sleep is greatly enhanced by proper nutrition. When you eat right, you aren't taking in a lot of harmful additives that interfere with hormonal performance and mental balance. The inevitable result is better sleep. Proper nutrition also contributes immeasurably to improved blood sugar control which goes a long way toward helping you sleep through the night without waking up.

Oxygen is present in proteins, fats, and carbs, but there is more of it in carbs than anywhere else in the diet. As mentioned above, complex carbohydrates are also the richest sources of nutrients.

Finally, how does nutrition help with exercise? The most obvious answer is that excellent nutrition is what provides the fuel and nutrients to move your body in the first place. Slightly less obvious is the fact that if your nutrition is inferior, you may not feel up to exercising at all. When nutrition is truly awful, you may not even be safe exercising. Just think of those athletes who appear to be in good shape, yet they have heart attacks or strokes during competition. I can almost guarantee that they had either an unknown genetic anomaly, or their nutrition wasn't what it should have been.

Sometimes it is possible for electrolytes such as potassium or magnesium to be so severely out of balance that strenuous exercise causes a dangerous situation. Drinking fresh juices is a great way to make sure that never happens. Fresh vegetable juices are loaded with good electrolytes.

We could do a similar analysis for all 7 Keys, but I think you are probably getting the idea by now that the synergy between these keys is tremendously significant. They are almost like dominoes in formation. If you take one out, the chain won't fall right.

Having analyzed the keys, let's apply them to a real-life situation and see how that synergy can help you with your health challenges.

Health challenge scenario

Let's say that you are having a persistent problem with indigestion—a very common problem in our culture. Does attitude have an impact on digestion? You bet it does! How you handle stress is of critical importance to your digestion.

Remember your grandparents saying it wasn't nice to discuss religion or politics over the supper table? They were right. When we argue or even carry on an intellectually challenging conversation, we're calling on one part of our nervous system. When we try to digest food we're using the other part. They can't both be dominant at the same time. When we eat on the run, or argue over dinner, or just maintain a high stress atmosphere around mealtimes we aren't putting our bodies in the right mode to digest food and the result is indigestion.

How about water? Does it affect digestion? Absolutely. Stomach acid is partly water. Dehydration impairs your ability to produce adequate stomach acid. While most people assume that indigestion is the result of excess stomach acid, the opposite is usually true. Insufficient acid production leads to incomplete digestion—the true cause of most people's burning sensations.

Another way water impacts digestion is a matter of timing. If you drink a lot of water with your meal, you dilute the stomach acid you produce and make it ineffective. It's best to drink your water between, not with, your meals.

How does elimination help a digestive disturbance? Remember the guy who went to the doctor and said, "Hey doc, it hurts when I do this." The doctor said, "Right, stop doing that. And pay the secretary on your way out." Eating rubbish is a great way to upset your digestive apple cart. Stop it! Hydrogenated oils, preservatives, flavorings, and colors weren't meant to be eaten, and they certainly don't do you any good.

We've all seen TV commercials in which somebody's trying to eat an enormous plate of chili dogs and he's feeling the pain. The understanding waitress hands him an anti-acid pill so he can finish his food. Next you'll see a commercial for the best-selling drug class in America—laxatives. It just proves my point: the Standard American Diet is so bad, we need drugs to force it in and more drugs to get it back out. When your belly aches in the middle of a meal or right after, it's not telling you to get a pill. It's telling you that you just made a bad food decision.

Sleep affects digestion pretty much the same way it affects all body systems. You need to sleep to repair things, including your digestive system. The lining of your digestive tract should be replaced entirely by new healthy cells every week or two. If you don't get your sleep, this process of renewal could be slowed down. Sleep also helps your nervous system function well. Your nervous system is largely responsible for the peristaltic motion of your digestive tract that keeps things moving along in a coordinated manner. If you lose coordination, you may end up with irritation, constipation, diarrhea, or all three.

When you sleep, your body releases growth hormone, which helps keep you in that anabolic state that favors healing for every cell in your body. Poor sleep keeps you in a prolonged stress response state—a catabolic state that favors degenerative disease. When stress-response hormones dominate your internal scene, your ability to control your blood sugar also suffers greatly.

Could oxygen possibly matter? Of course. Remember that all brain function is dependent on a ready supply of oxygen. That's why they worry about you not breathing for more than a minute or two—brain damage is imminent and unavoidable without oxygen. Your brain is a major coordinator for all body systems, including your digestive system.

Another factor worth mentioning is that when you breathe correctly, your nervous system is cued to go into the relaxed state that favors good digestion instead of the hyped up "fight the bear" kind of state you get into with shallow chest breathing. If your digestion is poor, doing the breathing exercise in chapter 5 right before you eat is a great way to press the reset button on your nervous system and get in "relax and digest mode."

Just think of a deer on a grassy hillside. If a wolf comes along, his nervous system switches gears instantly. He stops eating and runs. Have you ever seen a fleeing deer with a feed bag strapped on multitasking himself to safety? He obeys his body's design and does one thing at a time.

How does nutrition affect digestion? Several ways. Making good food choices begins with choosing to eat actual food—not chemicals and refined junk food. If you eat real food, your chances of being able to break it down and handle it properly go way up. If you eat real food in good combinations that's even better. For example, cantaloupe and pot roast do not go well together in your stomach.

Healthy food choices mean more fruits and veggies. More fruits and veggies mean more fiber. Fiber keeps things moving right in your gut. Fiber also feeds the beneficial bacteria in your gut. Although you can't digest fiber, the beneficial bacteria can, and when you feed them what they need, they express their gratitude by producing vitamins you need right there in your gut where you can absorb them.

On a deeper level still, good food directly provides the nutrients that your body needs to produce energy for you to live on and stomach acid to digest more food. It's cyclical. There are a variety of vitamins and minerals necessary to produce hydrochloric acid. B vitamins are among those, and the vast majority of people are rather low on B vitamins. Synthetic chemical factory replicas of B vitamins don't do the job so well, but a really good diet should supply enough B vitamins to keep things running smoothly if you aren't already grossly deficient.

How does exercise help your digestion? As mentioned before, exercise helps keep the motion going in your intestinal tract. It's possible to carry around in excess of 20 pounds of waste in your gut. It's not a pretty picture, but you need to know. The motion of your intestine is sequential, kind of like spectators doing the wave at a ball game. It's hard for them to do that while each spectator has a twenty pound package sitting on his lap. It's hard for your intestine to do the wave too. Vigorous activity helps shake things loose.

Exercise also encourages you to drink more water, which helps you make stomach acid and move out waste. Exercise also improves your anxiety and stress handling capacity so you're more relaxed at meal times. You sleep better after exercise so healing and cleansing are improved also.

You can see how everything is related. No key is isolated from the others and no one key works as well without the others. Health is a door with seven locks. Now, you have all 7 Keys.

Knowing is half the battle, but it isn't enough. Taking action can be difficult. I want to encourage you never to give up, no matter what. There will be setbacks, but the only way to fail is to stop trying. There is a reward for every improvement you make—even though you may not feel it or see it today. So many rewards come in the form of bad things that don't happen it's nearly impossible to fully appreciate them.

But don't forget—you do reap what you sow! There are lots of ways to use this information to make good changes in your life that will pay off down the road. How you handle it will depend somewhat on where you are now. If you have a very serious illness, you can't afford to dabble in a nine-year plan for personal improvement. You need to jump in with both feet and give yourself every possible advantage. If you are basically okay, you may have time to take it at a more comfortable pace.

In either case, help is always available. The fastest way to master anything is to find a mentor who has mastered it already. I work with a certain number of clients in person; people who are dedicated to becoming as healthy as they can by taking responsibility for their own care. They get lots of one-on-one personalized suggestions for how to make rapid progress in the 7 key areas to get their health on track.

If you'd rather read it or view it and try it on your own, visit my website regularly for new articles, newsletters, and more books and learning materials such as integrated programs that are planned for the near future. There are videos and audios on food preparation and other relevant topics already in the works too. Hope to see you soon at www.awesomehealthmakeover.com.

Live well!

Appendix A

Useful Lists and Acronyms

1 Equation for Total Health   H=7k

2 Primary Causes of All Disease
- Toxicity
- Deficiency

3 Ways to Find Nutrient Dense Foods in the Grocery Store
- Stay in the produce section or frozen vegetable aisle
- Shop by color
- Check the ANDI Score

4F Failing Foods
- Fried foods
- Fragmented / fortified foods
- Foods with a face
- Franken-foods

5-Part Process for Dealing with Children
- Enthusiasm
- Explanation
- Example
- Expectations
- Encouragement

6 (1) **PROVEN Dietary Guidelines**

P—Plant-sourced foods
R—Raw foods
O—Organic foods
V—Variety of foods
E—Enzyme-rich foods
N—Nutrient dense foods

6 (2) Pillars of AWESOME Nutrition
- Salads
- Smoothies and fresh fruits
- Soups
- Juices
- Healthy Starches
- Steamed / Sautéed Vegetables

7 Keys to AWESOME Health

A - Attitude
W - Water
E - Elimination
S - Sleep
O - Oxygen
M - Maximum nutrition
E - Exercise

References

1. Fereydoon Batmanghelidj, M.D., *Your Body's Many Cries for Water* (Vienna, VA: Global Health Solutions, 1995)

2. Joel Fuhrman, M.D., *Eat to Live* (Boston New York London: Little, Brown and Company, 2003)

3. William D. Holloway, Jr. and Herb Joiner-Bey, N.D., *Water–The Foundation of Youth, Health and Beauty* (New York, NY: IMPAKT Health, 2002) page 44

4. Joel Fuhrman, M.D., *Eat Right America* (USA: Nutritional Excellence, LLC, 2010

5. Phyllis Balch, CNC, and James Balch, M.D., *Prescription for Nutritional Healing,* Third Edition (New York: Penguin Putnam Inc., 2000) page 3

6. Dr. Henry Cloud and Dr. John Townsend, *Boundaries* (Grand Rapids, MI: Zondervan Publishing House, 1992)

7. T. Colin Campbell, PhD, with Thomas M. Campbell II *The China Study* (Dallas, TX, BenBella Books, 2005) pages 21 and 27

8. J. K. Rowling, *Harry Potter and the Half-Blood Prince* (New York: Arthur A. Levine Books an imprint of Scholastic Inc., 2005)

9. Jeffrey M. Smith, *Seeds of Deception* (Fairfield, IA: Yes! Books, 2003)

10. Jennifer Ragan
http://ezinearticles.com/?Not-So-Sweet---the-AverageAmerican-Consumes-150-170-Pounds-of-Sugar-Each-Year&id=2252026
(Last accessed April 2, 2012)
Jennifer Ragan's website: http://bamboocorefitness.com

11. United States Department of Agriculture (USDA)
http://www.fns.usda.gov/tn/Resources/Nibbles/healthful_choices.pdf
(Last accessed April 2, 2012)

12. Journal of Clinical Infectious Diseases
April 15, 2011
http://www.idsociety.org
(Last accessed April 2, 2012)

13. Hallelujah Acres
www.hacres.com

14. Herbert Fox, *Disease in Captive Wild Mammals and Birds* (Philadelphia, London and Chicago: J. B. Lippincott Company, 1923)

15. Quoted in an article titled "One Quarter Of U.S. Poultry And Meat Tainted With Resistant Bacteria" by Christian Nordqvist titled located at http://www.medicalnewstoday.com/articles/222552.php

16. Anthony Robbins, "A Personal Journal / Get the Edge" Multimedia Program. page 28

About the Author

Jana L. Fortner, N.D.

For more than twenty years, Jana Fortner has had a passion for helping people and an inability to tolerate human suffering. After experiencing health problems herself that conventional medicine failed to address, she became increasingly aware of the shortcomings in modern preventive care. Especially struck by the number of people who never recovered from cancer, she believed God must have provided a way out that was not widely known or not yet discovered. Not wanting to see herself or her family among the many victims, she began searching for a natural way to prevent and reverse disease at age 16 by taking classes in advanced anatomy and physiology. She went on to earn a degree in middle school math and social studies education from the University of Kentucky.

Having succeeded experimentally in correcting many of her own problems by reading and implementing dietary improvements, she was determined to find a natural solution when her first child was diagnosed with asthma at age three and was reacting badly to medications.

She used her knowledge of children and natural health to write a syndicated newspaper column, The Natural Mom, which was published for four years.

Desiring to further her education in natural health, she began taking classes at the Alternative Medicine College of Canada. She completed her N.D. through Trinity College of Natural Health and continues to attend accredited professional seminars regularly.

Several years ago, she opened the Nutritional Health Education Center in Danville, Kentucky, a natural health consulting and coaching practice where she continues helping clients reach their full health potential, naturally.

www.ingramcontent.com/pod-product-compliance
Lightning Source LLC
Chambersburg PA
CBHW070010300526
45794CB00001B/272